Medicine of the Future

Yann Meunier

Medicine of the Future

Risk Assessment, Elimination or Mitigation,
and Action Plans for 28 Diseases
and Medical Conditions

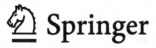

Yann Meunier
Hôpital Cochin
Paris
France

ISBN 978-3-319-36112-3   ISBN 978-3-319-07299-9   (eBook)
DOI 10.1007/978-3-319-07299-9
Springer Cham Heidelberg New York Dordrecht London

Printed on acid-free paper

Springer is part of Springer Science+Business Media (www.springer.com)

Foreword

You have addressed a wide variety of topics related to chronic disease. This is a list that is well beyond the menu of chronic disease management programs that I have seen. It seems to me that most of the patient visits to physician offices or clinics are for the conditions you have identified. Obviously, the expenditures for these conditions represent a huge financial cost burden to any nation, and the cost is likely to increase as populations age. Fortunately, most of the chronic conditions are caused by or are aggravated by an unhealthy lifestyle. In one sense, this is good news because changing one's lifestyle is both sustainable over time and less expensive to the medical care system. There may be additional chronic diseases for which you will need to develop new programs, but I see that as opportunity rather than deficiency in your planning. As you continue your work, more programs can be developed with the same attention to scientific best practice recommendations, and you will be able to reach a larger population.

You indicate in your request for my review that these materials contain state-of-the-art information for each disease/condition on genetic and biologic markers, personal and family medical history, demographics, and comorbidities. My review supports your contention that the information should not be considered as supplementary but instead significant to the medical evaluation, diagnosis, and recommendations offered to the patient. It seems to me that this is often a missing component to the delivery of medical care both in the US and in other countries. With this type of information, risk factors can be identified early and mitigated prior to unnecessary progression of the disease caused by lack of preventive tactics. This is the future of medicine, where the medical provider becomes a patient advocate for healthy lifestyle as a way of promoting health and preventing disease.

I know that you are an expert in the development of personal action plans, plans that are based in behavioral science and tactics that have demonstrated efficacy as well as sustained impact. As I read the action plans, I was impressed with the thoughtful content and, of equal importance, the processes that are recommended within the personal wellness plans. There is a subtle but extremely important shift in the relationship between physician and patient: one that sees the physician encouraging the patient to become an active participant in the health promotion/disease prevention strategy and one in which the patient now has adequate tools for assuming this responsibility. The medical outcome is likely to be favorably changed when the patient does this. The physician is working *with* the patient as an advocate, and it goes beyond the more typical medical model, which sees the physician working *for* the patient. This shift in paradigm is a significant benefit to patients, and when adopted as a population health strategy, the physician's role will become more important than is currently the case.

I believe that forward-thinking organizations and medical groups will find your document to be quite attractive. With medicine having such a long history where the doctor "treats" the patient with medicine or surgery while overlooking the essential root causes, I see your programs as being ambitious and I hope that you are successful. We need models such as this to demonstrate that lifestyle and the advocacy relationship between physician and patient are key to major breakthroughs in population health. I wish you much success. Wes

Wes Alles, PhD
Stanford University Prevention Research Center
Stanford University
Stanford, CA, USA

About the Author

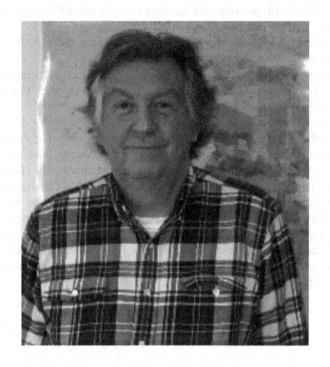

Yann Meunier, MD, was the director of International Corporate Affairs and Business Development for Stanford Hospital and Clinics and the director of the Stanford Health Promotion Network.

He was assistant professor in public health at Rene Descartes University in Paris, adjunct assistant professor of Medicine at George Washington University, and lecturer on "Urbanization and Public Health in Developing Countries" at the George Washington University Center for International Health.

He was a medical doctorate thesis director and advisor in various Paris universities on public health topics such as "Epidemiological Study and Screening for Cervix Cancer by PAP Smear in Lifou, New Caledonia."

As the chief medical officer for a US corporation in Papua New Guinea, he created and implemented a public health program for about 10,000 villagers in the Kutubu area of the Southern Highlands Province.

In Singapore, for a charity organization, he led a medical team pioneering public health programs for the Yi people in the Yunnan Province of China. As the first and only French private practitioner in the city-state, he addressed public health topics for the expatriate community such as: "Influence of Climate on Health," "Young People and HIV/AIDS," "Healthcare in Southeast Asia," "Malaria in Asia," and "The Use of Drugs and Alcohol by Teenagers."

As the first and only private practitioner in Lifou, New Caledonia, he wrote a report on public health priorities for the island, which incited the French government to tackle potable water and other sanitation issues.

He has field experience of HIV/AIDS, malaria, dengue fever, SARS, Japanese encephalitis, and meningitis.

He is widely published on Preventive Medicine matters such as "Struggle Against Cholera," "Precautions to Take Before Traveling to a Tropical Country," and "Hepatitis B: Who Must Be Immunized?"

He is editorial manager of the *American Journal of Preventive Medicine* and reviewer for the *Journal of Public Health, Scandinavian Journal of Public Health, Health Affairs, Journal of Public Health and Epidemiology*, and *International Journal of Collaborative Research on Internal Medicine and Public Health*.

Currently, he is the CEO of HealthConnect International LLC, a healthcare consulting company based in Silicon Valley, CA, and mentor in the Medscholars Research Fellowships Program at Stanford University School of Medicine.

He is honorary member of the Brazilian Academy of Medicine, associate member of the Academy of Medicine, Singapore, member of the International Academy of Fellows and Associates, Royal College of Physicians and Surgeons of Canada and fellow of the Australasian College of Tropical Medicine.

Acknowledgments

The author wishes to thank the following persons:

Wesley F. Alles, PhD
Director, Stanford Health Improvement Program–
Stanford Prevention Research Center, Stanford School of Medicine

John W. Farquhar, MD
Professor emeritus, Medicine, Stanford University
Emeritus faculty, Academic Council, Stanford University

Paul Wise, MD, PhD
Richard E. Behrman professor of Child and Health Society
Center for Health Policy/Center for Primary Care and Outcomes Research director
Core faculty member, Stanford University

Oscar Salvatierra, Jr., MD
Professor of surgery and pediatrics, active emeritus
Advising dean, Stanford University Medical Center, Stanford University School of Medicine

George W. Rutherford, MD, AM
Salvatore Pablo Lucia professor of Epidemiology,
Preventive Medicine, Pediatrics and History
Vice chair, Department of Epidemiology and Biostatistics
Director, Prevention and Public Health Group,
Global Health Sciences, University of California San Francisco

Marc Gentilini, MD
Professor emeritus in infectious and tropical diseases,
Pitié-Salpêtrière Hospital, Paris, France
Former president of the French Academy of Medicine
Former chair of the French Red Cross
President of the Water Academy

Luis Felippe de Queiros Mattoso, MD
Member of the Brazilian Academy of Medicine
Professor of radiology, Universidade do Estado de Rio de Janeiro, Brazil

Donald P. Francis, MD, DSc
Executive director at Global Solutions for Infectious Diseases

Many thanks to Dr. Patricia Patton for her unwavering support and for her inner and outer beauty.
Last but not least, this book is dedicated to *Sammy* the cat (aka Singapore Sling) who spent as much time cuddling by the computer as the author did researching and typing on it.

Contents

Introduction

We live in a time when healthcare costs are soaring worldwide. Healthcare systems of the future should be patient and not healthcare provider centered. The latter's primary role will be to empower patients to become fully in charge of their well-being so that they stay healthy as long as possible as opposed to seeing them mainly when they are sick nowadays.

This will also help delay or prevent the appearance of chronic diseases, which represent the bulk of healthcare and healthcare-related expenses in the current societal and economic environments. Indeed, for the most part, it will take heavy technology, which is the main driver of healthcare costs, out of the spending equation. Placing prevention at the core of the healthcare system will contain and hopefully reduce spending.

In order to achieve this mutation, healthcare providers will have first and foremost to inform healthy people about their risk profile qualitatively (for which diseases/medical conditions are they at risk?) and quantitatively (how high is the risk for each disease/medical condition?).

Medicine is only at the infancy stage of adopting really cost-effective prevention as the mainstay of healthcare. As a matter of fact, the bulk of patients in medical practices of the future will be healthy, and their main issue will be risk management. We are obviously a long way from reaching this situation. The healthcare field must morph from an essentially reactive discipline to a mainly proactive one. We have already used this novel approach with great success in smoking awareness/cessation campaigns and health promotion plans in specific environments. The positive outcome was mainly due to the fact that we knew health consequences and the cost of inaction. Going forward, generalizing this stance to all diseases and medical conditions is the key to productive healthcare management individually and collectively. The first step of prevention is risk assessment. It can be made at various levels: genetic, biochemical, serological, past medical history, family history, comorbidities, age, gender, ethnicity, nutrition, and lifestyle. They are all addressed in this book regarding 28 diseases and medical conditions to determine a risk profile for each individual. Recommendations are made to avoid, eliminate, or mitigate risks, and preventive measures are suggested concerning chemical compounds intake, lifestyle, and nutrition.

The next step is for physicians to establish, with their patients and taking into account their physical and human milieus (including enabling and hindrance factors), health action plans that will often rely on behavior change. The aggregation of science-based data should also enable practitioners to elaborate disease management programs with all individuals.

Furthermore, combined with using motivation assessment tools, evaluating readiness for change and developing and implementing these health promotion programs will facilitate the delivery of primary, secondary, and tertiary prevention initiatives at community levels. This book addresses essentially the individual level. Ultimately, patients are responsible for their own health and should be informed and invigorated to make the right choices.

In conceptualizing this book, my main drivers were to: (1) write a pamphlet taking the approach to each disease and medical condition as an argument toward a new attitude in dealing with them, (2) impart new knowledge and/or old knowledge in a new way, (3) provide a process template for dealing with diseases before they manifest themselves and possibly delay or prevent their emergence, and (4) hope that it will represent a beacon on the path to medicine of the future.

One fiction scenario that could become reality is the extension of individual lifespan by organ substitution. Based on thorough risk assessment, computer modeling and organ reconstitution using stem cells, organ failures could be predicted well before they happen and new organs readied as needed.

Right now a critical mass of novel mindset is needed if we want to improve healthcare delivery everywhere by adopting or imitating the new matrix I suggest. In doing so, we will avoid all the disastrous consequences of a collapse of the current healthcare model, which is inevitable despite measures taken and proposed.

Yann Meunier, MD

P.S.: The information included in this book is meant to be completed, updated, and expanded, particularly as genetic testing and biochemical and serological markers become more numerous, reliable, affordable, thorough, and widespread. Additionally, a large space is available for new risks to be discovered and for current ones to be better quantified. Thus, present preventive strategies will be improved and new ones created.

Chapter 1
Diseases and Medical Conditions

1.1 Abdominal Aortic Aneurysm

1.1.1 Risk Assessment and Prevention of Abdominal Aortic Aneurysm (AAA)

1.1.1.1 Risk Assessment

Genetic Markers

- People with a common variant in a gene known as DAB2IP on chromosome 9 have a significantly increased risk of developing AAA.
- There is evidence for genetic heterogeneity, and the presence of AAA suscepti- bility loci can be found on chromosomes 19q13 and 4q31. Please see Table 1.1.

Biochemical and Serological Markers

- People with lower HDL levels and higher LDL levels have an increased risk of developing AAA.
- People with higher creatinine levels have an increased risk of developing AAA. Please see Table 1.2.

Past Medical History

- People with a history of angina pectoris, coronary heart disease, and myocardial infarction have an increased risk of developing AAA.

Y. Meunier, *Medicine of the Future: Risk Assessment, Elimination or Mitigation, and Action Plans for 28 Diseases and Medical Conditions,* DOI 10.1007/978-3-319-07299-9_1, © Springer International Publishing Switzerland 2014

Table 1.1 Chromosomal loci-harboring genes for syndromic and nonsyndromic aortic aneurysms

Chromosomal region	Disease	Inheritance	OMIM ID	OMIM locus symbol	Gene
2q31	Ehlers–Danlos syndrome type IV	AD	130050	EDS4	COL3A1
3p22	TAAD	AD	608967	AAT3	TGFBR2
3p22	Loeys–Dietz syndrome	AD	609192	LDS	TGFBR2
4q31	AAA		609782	AAA2	
5q13–q14	TAAD	AD	607087	AAT2	
9q33–q34	TAAD	AD	610380	AAT5	TGFBR1
9q33–q34	Loeys–Dietz syndrome	AD	609192	LDS	TGFBR1
11q23.3–q24	TAAD	AD	607086	AAT1	
15q21.1	Marfan syndrome	AD	154700	MFS	FBN1
15q24–26	TAAD	AD		AAT6	
16p13.13–p13.12	TAAD with patent ductus arteriosus	AD	132900	AAT4	MYH11
19q13	AAA		609781	AAA1	

From: *Circulation* (2008) 117(2):243–252
All loci except the EDS4 and AAT5 were identified by DNA linkage studies with either family-based or "affected relative pair" approaches. For a complete list of the original studies, please see http://www.ncbi.nlm.nih.gov/entrez/query.fcgi?CMD=search&DB=OMIM. No genes harboring mutations in aneurysm patients in the AAA1, AAA2, AAT1, AAT2, or AAT6 loci have yet been identified. Official approved gene symbols were obtained from www.gene.ucl.ac.uk/nomenclature
OMIM Online Mendelian Inheritance in Man, *ID* identification, *AD* autosomal dominant, *COL3A1* gene symbol for type III procollagen, *TGFBR1* and *2* gene symbols for transforming growth factor-β receptors 1 and 2, and *MYH11* gene symbol for smooth muscle myosin heavy chain

Table 1.2 Markers of activity associated with AAA

Biological markers	Biological activity
Blood–wall interface	
Platelet activation	Thrombosis
Fibrin formation	Thrombosis
Matrix metalloproteinase 9	Neutrophil degranulation
Elastase/antielastase	Neutrophil degranulation
Myeloperoxidase	Neutrophil degranulation
Plasminogen activators	Fibrinolysis
Plasmin/antiplasmin	Fibrinolysis
D-Dimer	Fibrinolysis
Wall media	
Collagen peptides	Extracellular matrix degradation
Elastin peptides	Extracellular matrix degradation
Adventitia or wall media	
IL-6	Immunoinflammation
IL-8	Immunoinflammation
IFN-γ	Immunoinflammation
Osteopontin	Immunoinflammation
C-reactive protein	Immunoinflammation

From: *Nat Rev Cardiol* (2011) 8:338–347. doi:10.1038/nrcardio.2011.1
Abbreviations: *AAA* abdominal aortic aneurysm, *IFN* interferon, *IL* interleukin

Family History

- People who have a first-degree relative (parent, brother, sister) with AAA that required surgical repair have a 12-fold increased risk of developing AAA.

Comorbidities

- Inherited connective tissue disorders, most commonly Marfan syndrome and Ehlers–Danlos syndrome, increase the risk of developing AAA.
- Cystic medial necrosis increases the risk of developing AA.
- Arteritis increases the risk of developing AAA.
- Infected or mycotic aneurysm increases the risk of developing AAA.
- Pseudoaneurysms (false aneurysms involving adventitia and media but not the intimal wall of the aorta) occur with trauma and adjacently to prior aortic repairs, in which case they are termed "anastomotic." They increase the risk of developing AAA.
- Peripheral artery disease increases the risk of developing AAA.
- People with obesity have an increased risk of developing AAA.
- People with type 2 diabetes have an increased risk of developing AAA.
- People with high blood pressure have an increased risk of developing AAA.
- People with emphysema have an increased risk of developing AAA.
- People with arteriosclerosis have a strong risk of developing AAA.
- People with lower ankle–arm blood pressure ratio have an increased risk of developing AAA.
- People with higher maximum carotid stenosis have an increased risk of developing AAA.
- People with greater intima–media thickness of the internal carotid artery have an increased risk of developing AAA.
- Syphilis increases the risk of developing AAA.

Age/Gender/Ethnicity/Nutrition/Lifestyle

- AAA prevalence is 3–10 % for patients >50 years old in the Americas and Europe.
- Caucasians have a higher risk of developing AAA than blacks.
- Men have a higher risk of developing AAA than women (the ratio being between 2:1 and 6:1, respectively).
- Males over 65 have an increased risk of developing AAA.
- People who smoke (or have smoked) have an increased risk of developing AAA.
- Alcohol is a risk factor for developing AAA.
- Deficiency in vitamin B12, along with vitamins B6 and folate, may increase the risk of developing aneurysm.
- Copper deficiency has been associated with AAA.
- Greater height is associated with a higher risk of developing AAA.

Similarly:

- The risk of aneurysm rupture is higher in women (up to threefold higher in one study).

Recommendations

- Eliminate/avoid/attenuate risk factors, if possible (please see above and below).
- Men over 65 and under 75 who smoke or have smoked (at least 100 cigarettes in their lifetime) should be checked once a year by abdominal ultrasound.

1.1.1.2   Preventive Advice

Chemical

- Statins and some antibiotics may slow the growth of small aortic aneurysms.
- There is some evidence that losartan may prevent aneurysm formation.
- Vitamin E has been shown to inhibit the formation of AAA in mice.
- B12, along with vitamins B6 and folate supplements must be taken in case of deficiency.
- Copper should be taken if there is a deficiency.

Similarly:

- Caution must be taken with aspirin use in case of unruptured aneurysm (medical advice is needed).

Lifestyle

- Control blood pressure (use medications such as beta-blockers, if necessary).
- Control blood sugar.
- Get regular exercise (please see Sect. 2.1).
- Reduce stress (please see Sect. 2.2).
- Do not smoke/quit smoking or chewing tobacco (please see Sect. 2.3).

Nutrition

- Reduce cholesterol and fat in the diet (please see Sect. 2.7). The Stanford University Health Improvement Program recommends the Mediterranean diet for cholesterol control.
- Drink alcohol with moderation (please see Sect. 2.4).

1.2 Alzheimer's Disease

1.2.1 Risk Assessment and Prevention of Alzheimer's Disease (AD)

1.2.1.1 Risk Assessment

Genetic Markers

- Scientists have discovered variations that directly cause Alzheimer's disease in the genes coding three proteins: amyloid precursor protein (APP), presenilin-1 (PS-1), and presenilin-2 (PS-2). When Alzheimer's disease is caused by these deterministic variations, it is called "autosomal dominant Alzheimer's disease (ADAD)" or "familial Alzheimer's disease," and many family members in multiple generations are affected. Their symptoms nearly always develop before age 60 and may appear as early as in someone's 30s or 40s.
- People with the risk gene apolipoprotein E-e4 (ApoE-e4) have an increased risk of developing AD.
- Half the people with two ApoE4 genes will develop Alzheimer's, compared with about one-fourth of people with one copy and 10 % of people with no copies.
- People with two copies also develop symptoms earlier, around age 68, years before most people with one copy and more than a decade before most people without the gene.
- People with two ApoE4 genes make up only about 3 % of the population.
- The ApoE genotype-specific effects on Alzheimer's disease vary by age and sex. The epsilon 4 allele has a stronger risk effect in men, and the epsilon 2 allele confers a protective effect only in younger-old people.
- For ApoE genotype variant frequencies and ethnicity, please see Table 1.3.
- For early-onset familial Alzheimer's disease (EOFAD), please see Tables 1.4 and 1.5.

Table 1.3 ApoE variant frequencies

Genotype	European ethnicity (%)	African American ethnicity (%)	East Asian ethnicity (%)
ε2/ε2	0.3	0.4	0.2
ε2/ε3	10.8	13.3	7.9
ε3/ε3	57.4	41.7	74.6
ε2/ε4	2.2	2.4	0.9
ε3/ε4	24.0	34.1	15.4
ε4/ε4	2.9	3.6	1.0

From: *Arch Neurol* (2011) 68(12):1569–1579 and *Hum Mol Genet* (2006) 15(13):2170–2182

Table 1.4 EOFAD molecular genetics

Locus name	Proportion of EOFAD	Gene symbol	Protein name	Test availability
AD3	20–70 %	*PSEN1*	Presenilin-1	Clinical
AD1	10–15 %	*APP*	Amyloid beta A4 protein	Clinical
AD4	Rare	*PSEN2*	Presenilin-2	Clinical

Table 1.5 Summary of molecular genetic testing used in early-onset familial Alzheimer's disease

Gene symbol	Proportion of EOFAD attributed to mutations in this gene (%)	Test method	Mutations detected	Mutation detection frequency by gene and test method	Test avail-ability
PSEN1	30–70	Targeted mutation analysis	4,555-bp deletion of exon 9 (Finnish founder mutation)	100 % for the targeted mutation	Clinical
		Sequence analysis	Sequence variants	~98 %	
		Deletion/ duplication analysis	Partial- and whole-gene deletions, including exon 9 Finnish founder deletion	100 % for deletions, which are rare	
PSEN2	<5	Sequence analysis	Sequence variants	~100 %	Clinical
APP	10–15	Sequence analysis/ mutation scanning 6 of exons 16 and 17	Sequence variants in exons 16 and 17	99 %	Clinical
		Deletion/ duplication analysis 5	Partial- and whole-gene duplications	100 % for the targeted duplication	

From: http://www.ncbi.nlm.nih.gov/books/NBK1236/

Biochemical and Serological Markers

- ApoE in the blood is a risk factor for developing AD.
- People with high cholesterol have an increased risk of developing AD.
- Other biological markers of AD can be found (1) in the cerebrospinal fluid (CSF), (2) as peripheral tissue markers, and (3) through pharmacological and neuroendocrine probes. Their type should be chosen and results analyzed by the physicians who request them. Please see Table 1.6.

Table 1.6 Internationally established biomarkers in CSF used to diagnose AD

Biomarker	Controls (pg/ml)	AD (pg/ml)
Aβ(1–42)	794 ± 20	<500*
Total tau	136 ± 89 (21–50 years)	a
	243 ± 127 (51–70 years)	>450
	341 ± 171 (>71 years)	>600*
Phospho-tau-181	23 ± 2	>60*

From: *Trends Biotechnol* (2011) 29(1):26–32
Data obtained using the Innogenetics single 96-well ELISA kits
*$p<0.001$
aThis is not relevant for sporadic AD, because it is only for patients >60 years of age

Past Medical History

- People with mild cognitive impairment are more likely to develop AD.
- Having high blood pressure for a long time increases the risk of developing AD.
- A positive past medical history of head trauma increases the risk of developing AD.

Family History

- The risk of developing AD appears to be higher if a first-degree relative has the disease.

Comorbidities

- Down syndrome is a risk factor for AD.
- People at risk for heart disease have an increased risk of developing AD.
- People with poorly controlled diabetes have an increased risk of developing AD.
- Obese people have an increased risk of developing AD.

Age/Gender/Ethnicity/Nutrition/Lifestyle

- The older people get, the higher the risk for developing AD. After age 65, the risk of developing the disease doubles about every 5 years.
- After age 85, the risk of developing AD reaches nearly 50 %.
- Women are more likely than men to develop AD, partly because they live longer.
- Japanese-American men have significantly higher rates of Alzheimer's disease than men of comparable age in Japan.

- There are higher rates of AD among African Americans than among Africans.
- Lack of involvement in mentally and socially stimulating activities increases the risk of developing AD.
- People who do not exercise have an increased risk of developing AD.
- People who smoke have an increased risk of developing AD.

Recommendations

- Eliminate/avoid/attenuate risk factors, if possible.
- When there is a suspicion of AD, a full set of tests should be performed, including physical and neurological exams, lab tests, mental status tests, neuropsychological tests, and brain imaging (CT/MRI/PET).

1.2.1.2   Preventive Advice

Chemical

- Statins, niacin, and other drugs can control cholesterol.
- Various medications can control blood pressure.
- Various medications can control blood sugar.
- Omega-3 fatty acids bring possible benefits to cognitive health.
- Ginkgo biloba has been shown to induce a small improvement in cognitive functions.

Lifestyle

- Exercise regularly (please see Sect. 2.1).
- Do not smoke/stop smoking or chewing tobacco (please see Sect. 2.3).
- Control blood pressure.
- Control cholesterol, if possible without drugs (please see Sect. 2.7).
- Control blood sugar levels and prevent diabetes, if possible without drugs (please see Sect. 2.8).
- Avoid head trauma and protect head (using helmets) when they may happen.
- Engage socially.
- Participate in intellectually stimulating activities.

Nutrition

- A diet low in fat, high in fiber, and rich in fruits and vegetables may help protect cognitive health.
- Drink alcohol with moderation (please see Sect. 2.4).

1.3   Atrial Fibrillation

1.3.1   Risk Assessment and Prevention of Atrial Fibrillation (A-fib)

1.3.1.1   Risk Assessment

Genetic Markers

- 34 out of 100 men of European ethnicity who share Greg Mendel (Dad)'s genotype will get A-fib before reaching 79 years of age.
- On chromosome e4q25, the marker rs2200733 SNP might affect the closest gene, called PITX2, which encodes a transcription factor known to be involved in heart development. The riskier version of this SNP might perturb the normal structure of the heart and thus predispose a person to A-fib. Another SNP near PITX2 has also been associated with atrial fibrillation in people with Asian and European ancestry.
- Please see the table in *European Journal of Human Genetics* (10 July 2013) doi:10.1038/ejhg.2013.139, via the following link: http://www.nature.com/ejhg/journal/v22/n3/full/ejhg2013139a.html.

Biochemical and Serological Markers

- Please see Table 1.7, for biomarkers and arrhythmias.

Past Medical History

The following diseases/conditions can cause A-fib:
- High blood pressure
- High pulse pressure
- Coronary disease and heart attacks
- Abnormal heart valves (particularly the mitral valve)
- Congenital heart defects
- Overactive thyroid gland or other metabolic imbalances
- Sick sinus syndrome
- Asthma
- COPD
- Previous heart surgery (including for congenital heart disease)
- Viral infections
- Stress due to surgery, pneumonia, or other illnesses
- Sleep apnea
- Hyperthyroidism

Table 1.7 Biomarkers and arrhythmias

		Clinical associations	
Biomarker	Associated mechanism	Atrial fibrillation	Ventricular tachyarrhythmias
BNP	Increased myocardial tension	Predict incident AF in general population	Risk factor for SCD in women
NT-pro-BNP		Increased serum levels in AF compared to sinus rhythm	Risk factor for SCD in heart failure
			Associated with VT 1 year post-MI
			Associated with ICD shocks
CRP	Inflammation	Risk factor for incident AF in general population	Risk factor for SCD in healthy individuals
	Oxidative stress		
	Apoptosis	Higher levels in AF	
DROM	Oxidative stress	Serum levels higher in AF compared to sinus rhythm	
Aldosterone	Increased myocardial tension	Increased levels in AF	Aldosterone inhibition decreases SCD in heart failure
	Fibrosis	Decreases after restoration to sinus rhythm	
	Electrical remodeling		
Cystatin C	Marker for glomerular filtration rate	Risk factor for AF in general population	Risk factor for SCD in general population
Trans-fatty acid	Inflammation		Risk factor for SCD
	Endothelial dysfunction		

From: *Cardiovasc Ther* (2012) 30(2):e74–e80

Family History

- The heritability of atrial fibrillation is estimated at 62 %.

Comorbidities

- Rheumatic fever and endocarditis increase the risk of developing A-fib.
- Peri-/myocarditis and cardiomyopathy increase the risk of developing A-fib.
- Heart failure increases the risk of developing A-fib.
- Pneumonia increases the risk of developing A-fib.
- Pulmonary embolism increases the risk of developing A-fib.

- Obesity increases the risk of developing A-fib.
- Diabetes increases the risk of developing A-fib.
- Pheochromocytoma increases the risk of developing A-fib.
- Chronic kidney disease increases the risk of developing A-fib.
- Fever increases the risk of developing A-fib.
- Stress increases the risk of developing A-fib.
- Adrenergic stimulation increases the risk of developing A-fib.
- Vagal stimulation increases the risk of developing A-fib.
- Hyper- or hypokalemia increases the risk of developing A-fib.

Similarly:

- A-fib is a risk factor for stroke.

Age/Gender/Ethnicity/Nutrition/Lifestyle

- A-fib is considerably more common among men than women.
- The risk of A-fib increases with age, particularly after 60.
- Caucasians have an increased risk of developing A-fib.
- Drinking alcohol can trigger an episode of atrial fibrillation in some people. Binge drinking—five drinks in 2 h for men or four drinks for women—may create a higher risk of developing A-fib.
- Smoking increases the risk of developing A-fib.
- High-endurance sport increases the risk of developing A-fib.
- The use of stimulants such as amphetamines and decongestants that contain stimulants (particularly pseudoephedrine), illegal drugs (cocaine, methamphetamines), and excessive nicotine or caffeine increases the risk of developing A-fib.
- The use of some prescription medicines, such as albuterol or theophylline, increases the risk of developing A-fib.
- Many dietary supplements can stimulate heart tissues and are not advised such as tyrosine, phenylalanine, SAM-e, alpha-lipoic acid, ginseng, tongkat ali, and yohimbe.
- Magnesium deficiency induces arrhythmias, including A-fib.
- High doses of vitamin D could also be a risk factor for developing A-fib.

Recommendations

- Eliminate/avoid/attenuate risk factors, if possible (please see above).
- Treat underlying conditions.
- Check heartbeat regularly.

1.3.1.2   Preventive Advice

Chemical

- In people with A-fib, anti-arrhythmic medications are prescribed to prevent episodes of A-fib. Commonly used medications include:
  - Amiodarone
  - Dronedarone
  - Propafenone
  - Sotalol
  - Dofetilide
  - Flecainide

  (Similarly, pacemakers are sometimes needed to prevent A-fib.)
- Take antibiotics to prevent endocarditis, if necessary.
- Vitamin C may be helpful.
- Magnesium supplement is needed when there is a deficiency.
- Correct hyper- or hypokalemia.

Lifestyle

- Engage in physical activity (please see Sect. 2.1), but be careful with high-endurance sport, if at risk for A-fib (check with your physician).
- Manage stress (please see Sect. 2.2).
- Do not smoke/quit smoking or chewing tobacco (please see Sect. 2.3).
- Control weight and, if necessary, lose weight by increasing caloric output through exercising and decreasing caloric intake through dieting.
- Control blood pressure.

Nutrition

- Avoid some medicines, if possible and if at risk (please see above), and stimulants—such as caffeine or nicotine.
- Drink alcohol with moderation (please see Sect. 2.4).
- Eat heart-healthy foods. The Stanford University Health Improvement Program recommends the Mediterranean diet (please see Sect. 2.7).
- Use less salt, which helps to lower blood pressure.
- Fish oils reduce arrhythmias, including A-fib.

1.4   Brain Aneurysm

1.4.1   Risk Assessment and Prevention of Brain Aneurysm

1.4.1.1   Risk Assessment

Genetic Markers

- rs10757278-G is associated with intracranial aneurysm. Compared to the AG genotype, the GG genotype increases a person's odds of having an intracranial aneurysm by about 1.3 times, while the AA genotype decreases a person's odds by about 1.3 times as well. People with a G at both copies have 1.54 times the odds compared to those with the AA genotype.
- Each G at rs1429412 increases a person's chance of having a brain or intracranial aneurysm.
- rs10958409 increases a person's chance of having a brain, or intracranial, aneurysm. People with the AG genotype at the SNP have 1.42 times the odds of having a brain aneurysm compared to those with the GG genotype. People with an A at both copies have 1.83 times the odds compared to those with the GG genotype.
- Each G at rs700675 increases a person's chance of having a brain, or intracranial, aneurysm. People with the AA genotype at the SNP have 0.91 times the odds of having an intracranial aneurysm compared to those with the AG genotype. People with a G at both copies have 1.44 times the odds compared to those with the AG genotype.

SNPs associated with brain aneurysm

SNP	Risk version	Effect (increase in odds per copy compared to two copies of non-risk version)
rs12413409	G	1.29
rs9315204	T	1.20
rs11661542	C	1.22

Similarly:

- People with eNOS genetic polymorphisms such as intron-4 27 base pair, variable number of tandem repeats (27 VNTR), promoter single-nucleotide polymorphism (T-786C SNP), and exon-7 SNP (G894T SNP) are ten times more likely to suffer a stroke from a ruptured brain aneurysm than people who have aneurysms but lack these key genetic variations.

Biochemical and Serological Markers

The following increases the risk of developing brain aneurysm:

- Alpha-glucosidase deficiency
- Alpha 1-antitrypsin deficiency
- Elevated serum elastase
- Hypercholesterolemia
- Lower estrogen levels after menopause

Past Medical History

- People born with the following conditions have an increased risk of developing brain aneurysms:

  - Inherited connective tissue disorders, such as type IV Ehlers–Danlos syndrome
  - Polycystic kidney disease
  - Coarctation of the aorta
  - Cerebral arteriovenous malformation

- People who had a head injury have an increased risk of developing brain aneurysms.
- People who had certain blood infections have an increased risk of developing brain aneurysms.
- People who had a brain aneurysm are more likely to have another one.

Family History

- People who have a first-degree relative with a history of brain aneurysm have an increased risk of developing the disease.
- Autosomal dominant polycystic kidney disease in the family increases the risk of developing brain aneurysm.
- Hereditary hemorrhagic telangiectasias increase the risk of developing brain aneurysm.

Comorbidities

- Aneurysm in other vessels increases the risk of developing brain aneurysm.
- People with hypertension have an increased risk of developing brain aneurysm.
- Arteriosclerosis increases the risk of developing brain aneurysm.
- Diabetes increases the risk of developing brain aneurysm.

- Neurofibromatosis type 1 increases the risk of developing brain aneurysm.
- Fibromuscular dysplasia increases the risk of developing brain aneurysm.
- Tuberous sclerosis increases the risk of developing brain aneurysm.
- Pheochromocytoma increases the risk of developing brain aneurysm.
- Klinefelter syndrome increases the risk of developing brain aneurysm.
- Noonan syndrome increases the risk of developing brain aneurysm.
- Infection of vessel walls increases the risk of developing brain aneurysm.
- Intracranial neoplasm increases the risk of developing brain aneurysm.
- Intracranial neoplastic emboli increase the risk of developing brain aneurysm.

Age/Gender/Ethnicity/Nutrition/Lifestyle

- Aneurysms occur in all age groups, but the incidence increases steadily for individuals ages 25 and older.
- Aneurysms are most prevalent in people ages 50–60.
- Aneurysms are about three times more prevalent in women.
- People who smoke (or have smoked) have an increased risk of developing brain aneurysm.
- Heavy alcohol consumption increases the risk of developing brain aneurysm.
- Drug abuse, particularly of cocaine or amphetamines, increases the risk of developing brain aneurysm.
- Oral contraceptive use increases the risk of developing brain aneurysm.
- Deficiency in vitamin B12, along with vitamins B6 and folate, may increase the risk of developing brain aneurysm.
- Copper deficiency has been associated with aneurysms.

  Similarly:

- African Americans are more likely than whites to have ruptured brain aneurysms.

Recommendations

- Eliminate/avoid/attenuate risk factors, if possible (please see above and below).

1.4.1.2   Preventive Advice

Chemical

- There is some evidence that losartan may prevent aneurysm formation.
- Copper should be taken if there is a deficiency.
- Vitamin B12, vitamin B6, and folate supplements should be taken if there is a deficiency.

Similarly:

- Caution must be taken with aspirin use in case of unruptured brain aneurysm (medical advice is needed).

Lifestyle

- Adjust exercise and avoid straining (please see Sect. 2.1).
- Control blood pressure regularly.
- Reduce stress (please see Sect. 2.2).
- Do not smoke/quit smoking or chewing tobacco (please see Sect. 2.3).
- Limit caffeine intake.
- Do not use recreational drugs, in particular cocaine.

Nutrition

- Control cholesterol (please see Sect. 2.7).
- Drink alcohol with moderation (please see Sect. 2.4).

1.5   Breast Cancer

1.5.1   Risk Assessment and Prevention of Breast Cancer

1.5.1.1   Risk Assessment

Genetic Markers

- Women with the following genetic markers BRCA1 or BRCA2 mutation/ATM/ CHEK2/p53/PTEN have a highly increased risk of developing breast cancer.
- Women with certain BRCA1 mutations have about a 65 % lifetime risk of getting breast cancer.
- Women with a DNA variation on a gene locus located on the long arm of chromosome 6 are at a 1.4 times greater risk of developing breast cancer compared to those without the variation.
- Women with SNPs in the FGFR1 and TNRC9 genes, as well as a third SNP on chromosome 2, have an associated overall increase in risk of developing breast cancer.
- Women under 70 years of age with the highest polygenic risk scores have double the breast cancer risk (8.8 % compared to 4.4 % in women with the lowest polygenic scores).
- Several SNPs are associates with breast cancer. Please see Table 1.8.

Table 1.8 Comparison between the observed prevalence of known SNPs in 17 studied breast cancer samples and exome sequencing project

| Gene | 17 breast cancer samples | | | | ESP | | | | Chi-square test | | | | HapMap | | | | AA change | Polyphen score |
	#Samples	#Var alleles	#Ref alleles	Var/Ref alleles	#Var alleles	#Ref alleles	Var/Ref alleles	FREQ 17/FREQ ESP	Value	p	Yates value	Yates p	Afr	Eur	Asia	rsID		
HOOK2	3	6	28	0.21	8	12,136	0.001	325.1	912	0	766	0	0	0	7.3	2305376	G10R	0.99
ANTXR1	3	3	31	0.10	21	12,903	0.002	59.5	138	0	95	0	NA	NA	NA	28365986	R7K	0.009
MCOLN1	3	4	30	0.13	46	12,960	0.004	37.6	115	0	88	0	NA	NA	NA	73003348	T261M	0.614
C3orf17	3	4	30	0.13	65	12,925	0.005	26.5	82	0	62	0	NA	NA	NA	115971253	V297I	0.117
TNKS1BP1	5	6	28	0.21	182	12,808	0.014	15.1	63	0	52	0	NA	NA	NA	34448143	A100P	0.194
PLEC	4	6	28	0.21	185	12,391	0.015	14.4	59	0	49	0	NA	NA	NA	3135103	R569Q	0.993
DDX18	3	4	30	0.13	93	12,913	0.007	18.5	56	0	42	0	NA	NA	NA	61755349	V371I	0.011
APIM2	3	3	31	0.10	52	12,238	0.004	22.8	54	0	37	0	NA	NA	NA	34276903	Y85C	0.998
GEMIN4	3	6	28	0.21	297	12,201	0.024	8.8	33	0	27	0	NA	NA	NA	191778127	H873Q	0
LY75	5	8	26	0.31	658	12,348	0.053	5.8	24	0	20	0	NA	NA	NA	35941588	T1393I	0.435
TXNDC5	4	5	29	0.17	289	10,583	0.027	6.3	18.8	0.00001	14.4	0.0001	NA	NA	NA	183777097	P49S	0
HIST1H1B	6	6	28	0.21	512	12,494	0.041	5.2	16.7	0.00004	13.3	0.0003	0	7.5	0	34144478	A211T	0.404
IMPACT	8	11	23	0.48	1,602	11,404	0.140	3.4	12.5	0.0004	10.8	0.001	4.3	16.9	2.2	582234	D125E	0.001
AKAP9	7	9	25	0.36	1,229	11,777	0.104	3.4	11.4	0.0007	9.5	0.002	1.7	15	0.6	35759833	K2476R	0.001
QRSL1	3	5	29	0.17	456	12,550	0.036	4.7	12.5	0.0004	9.4	0.002	0	5	5.6	34221917	N263S	0.593
DSG2	6	7	27	0.26	759	11,175	0.068	3.8	11.5	0.0007	9.2	0.002	0	9.9	0.2	2230234	I293V	0.99
HLA-DRB5	6	10	24	0.42	1,288	10,016	0.129	3.2	10.9	0.001	9.2	0.002	NA	NA	NA	112872773	V209L	0
JRK	4	5	29	0.17	459	12,219	0.038	4.6	11.9	0.0006	8.9	0.002	NA	NA	NA	34288113	T30M	0.988
LAPTM5	11	14	20	0.70	2,541	10,465	0.243	2.9	10.1	0.001	8.8	0.003	2.5	25.8	7.2	35351292	R226K	0.002
DDRGK1	8	11	23	0.48	1,762	11,244	0.157	3.1	10.2	0.001	8.7	0.003	0	19.2	0	11591	A303T	0.004
KIF20B	7	12	22	0.55	2,044	10,952	0.187	2.9	9.8	0.001	8.4	0.004	2.5	26.9	37.9	1129777	A50G	0.918
GLB1	4	6	28	0.21	637	11,695	0.054	3.9	10.7	0.001	8.3	0.004	NA	NA	NA	73826339	S401G	0.001
WDR55	5	7	27	0.26	873	12,133	0.072	3.6	10.4	0.001	8.3	0.004	NA	NA	NA	35983033	Y235C	0.998

(continued)

Table 1.8 (continued)

Gene	#Samples	#Var alleles	#Ref alleles	Var/Ref Ref alleles	#Var alleles	#Ref alleles	Var/Ref Ref alleles	FREQ 17/ FREQ ESP	Value	p	Yates value	Yates p	Afr	Eur	Asia	rsID	AA change	Polyphen score
		17 breast cancer samples			ESP				Chi-square test				HapMap					
THUMPD3	8	10	24	0.42	1,564	11,442	0.137	3.0	9.7	0.001	8.1	0.004	4.3	18.9	7.8	1129174	R459Q	0.056
NLRP2	8	14	20	0.70	2,629	10,377	0.253	2.8	9.2	0.002	8	0.005	NA	NA	NA	34804158	T529A	0
XPO5	4	6	28	0.21	645	11,467	0.056	3.8	10.1	0.001	7.9	0.005	0	14.2	0	34324334	S241N	0.002
RRS1	3	4	30	0.13	374	12,560	0.030	4.5	9.4	0.002	6.6	0.01	NA	4.1	20.4	3739336	R191L	0.999
PLSCR1	6	6	28	0.21	770	12,236	0.063	3.4	8.3	0.004	6.4	0.01	NA	8.3	3.1	343320	H262Y	0.945
PTPN12	10	12	22	0.55	2,252	10,754	0.209	2.6	7.6	0.005	6.4	0.01	19.7	11.3	29.8	3750050	T573A	0.001
REV3L	4	6	28	0.21	789	12,215	0.065	3.3	7.9	0.004	6	0.01	3.8	4.1	0	458017	Y1156C	0.002
ERBB2IP	7	9	25	0.36	1,498	11,506	0.130	2.8	7.4	0.006	6	0.01	0	17.8	8.1	3213837	S274L	0.024
SHARPIN	4	4	30	0.13	401	12,255	0.033	4.1	8.1	0.004	5.6	0.02	NA	NA	NA	34674752	P294S	0.447
KIAA1755	10	19	15	1.27	4,605	8,401	0.548	2.3	6.2	0.01	5.4	0.02	10.8	47.5	38.8	3746471	R1045W	0.003
SEC63	3	4	30	0.13	427	12,579	0.034	3.9	7.6	0.006	5.2	0.02	NA	NA	NA	17854547	V556I	0.203
LAMC2	4	6	28	0.21	848	12,158	0.070	3.1	6.9	0.009	5.2	0.02	0	9.9	0.2	11586699	T124M	0.999
ZNF880	4	7	27	0.26	376	4,190	0.090	2.9	6.7	0.009	5.2	0.02	NA	NA	NA	14048	V12M	0.999
IGFBP7	7	8	26	0.31	640	5,676	0.113	2.7	6.6	0.01	5.2	0.02	NA	NA	NA	11573021	L11F	0.005
PHF3	3	3	31	0.10	255	12,751	0.020	4.8	8.2	0.04	5.1	0.02	NA	NA	NA	34288820	V525I	0.972
KIAA0232	3	4	30	0.13	395	11,489	0.034	3.9	7.5	0.006	5.1	0.02	NA	NA	NA	116439703	P1138S	0.22
PJA1	7	11	23	0.48	1,742	8,821	0.197	2.4	6.2	0.01	5.1	0.02	12.5	24.6	12.5	11539157	E606D	0.992
PRCP	3	3	31	0.10	265	12,741	0.021	4.7	7.8	0.005	4.8	0.03	NA	NA	NA	2228312	T465S	0.021
MXRA5	14	23	11	2.09	5,006	5,557	0.901	2.3	5.6	0.02	4.8	0.03	22	27.6	34.9	1974522	P1665S	0.689
PARP14	7	7	27	0.26	1,022	10,826	0.094	2.7	6.1	0.01	4.7	0.03	4	7.6	10.9	13093808	A561E	0.972
EML4	12	15	19	0.79	3,414	9,592	0.356	2.2	6.6	0.02	4.7	0.03	11.7	26.7	43.9	28651764	K398R	0.003
ACOX1	13	24	10	2.40	6,616	6,390	1.035	2.3	5.3	0.02	4.5	0.03	13.6	34.9	29	1135640	I312M	0.007
SP110	3	6	28	0.21	928	12,078	0.077	2.8	5.6	0.01	4.16	0.04	0	9	4	11556887	A128V	0.999

PPL	12	20	14	1.43	5,261	7,733	0.680	2.1	4.7	0.03	4	0.05	0	47.5	30.4	2037912	Q1573E	0.994
TBL2	3	4	30	0.13	489	12,517	0.039	3.4	5.9	0.01	3.9	0.05	NA	3.1	NA	35607697	V345I	0.969
ZBTB45	3	4	30	0.13	491	12,511	0.039	3.4	5.9	0.01	3.9	0.05	NA	NA	NA	35430780	D293E	0
TMEM106C	4	6	28	0.21	962	12,044	0.080	2.7	5.1	0.02	3.8	0.05	0	11.2	40.4	2286025	S175F	0.985

From: *Sci Rep* 3, Article number: 2256. doi:10.1038/srep02256, published on 25 July 2013

Presented above are the top 50 variants showing higher prevalence among the 17 samples. The variants are sorted according to descending chi-square value. High Polyphen score indicates high probability of the variant to alter the protein function

Biochemical and Serological Markers

- High levels of blood androgens (postmenopause) moderately increase the risk of developing breast cancer.
- High levels of blood estrogens increase the risk of developing breast cancer (pre and post menopause).
- IGF-1 elevated levels (premenopause) moderately increase the risk of developing breast cancer.
- Prognostic factors and proangiogenic and anti-angiogenic proteins are in Tables 1.9 and 1.10.

Table 1.9 Well-established and investigational prognostic factors in breast cancer

Well established	Investigational
Ki-67	pS2
Estrogen receptor	Mitosin
Progesterone receptor	Epidermal growth factor receptor
HER-2	Insulin-like growth factors
	Apoptosis-related proteins
	Cell cycle molecules
	Plasminogen activators and inhibitors
	Angiogenesis-related proteins

Table 1.10 Proangiogenic and anti-angiogenic proteins

Proangiogenic	Anti-angiogenic
Vascular endothelial growth factor	Angiostatin
Angiogenin	Endostatin
Angiopoetin-1	Interferon (alpha, beta)
Del-1	Interleukin-12
Fibroblast growth factors	2-Methoxyestradiol
Follistatin	Platelet factor 4
Interleukin-8	Thrombospondin
Leptin	CD59 complement fragment
Placental growth factor	Heparinases
Platelet-derived endothelial growth factor	*Tissue inhibitors of metalloproteinases*
Pleiotrophin	Vasostatin
Transforming growth factor-alpha	16 kDa prolactin fragment
Transforming growth factor-beta	
Tumor necrosis factor	
Vascular endothelial growth factor	
Hepatocyte growth factor	
Nitric oxide	
Erucamide	
Urokinase plasminogen activator	

From: *Breast Cancer Res* (2004) 6:109–118. doi:10.1186/bc

Past Medical History

- High breast density strongly increases the risk of developing breast cancer.
- Radiation therapy during youth strongly increases the risk of developing breast cancer.
- Having no pregnancies moderately increases the risk of developing breast cancer.
- Having a first pregnancy after 35 moderately increases the risk of developing breast cancer.
- High bone density moderately increases the risk of developing breast cancer.
- Long-term HRT with estrogen + progestin increases the risk of developing breast cancer.
- Having first menses before 12 increases the risk of developing breast cancer.
- Having menopause after 50 increases the risk of developing breast cancer.
- Natural or herbal hormones increase the risk of developing breast cancer.
- DES exposure increases the risk of developing breast cancer.
- Weight gain postmenopause weakly increases the risk of developing breast cancer.
- Radiation therapy to the lungs may increase the risk of developing breast cancer.
- Overweight premenopause weakly decreases the risk of developing breast cancer.

Family History

- People with a positive family history of breast cancer have an increased risk of developing breast cancer, and it is worse if:
  - It appeared in the mother or a sister before menopause.
  - Two or more cancers can be found in the family.
- However, in over 70 % of cases of breast cancer, there is no positive family history.

Comorbidities

- Lobular carcinoma in situ strongly increases the risk of developing breast cancer.
- The presence of proliferative breast lesions (with or without atypia) increases the risk of developing breast cancer: strongly for atypical hyperplasia and moderately for usual hyperplasia.
- Cancer in one breast increases the risk of developing breast cancer in the other.
- Uterus cancer increases the risk of developing breast cancer.
- Colon cancer increases the risk of developing breast cancer.
- Ovarian cancer increases the risk of developing breast cancer.

Age/Gender/Ethnicity/Nutrition/Lifestyle

- In the United States, 1/8 of women will develop breast cancer.
- Caucasians have a higher risk of developing breast cancer.
- Ashkenazi Jewish heritage weakly increases the risk of developing breast cancer.
- Above-average height weakly increases the risk of developing breast cancer.
- Upper middle class status weakly increases the risk of developing breast cancer.
- Alcohol intake increases the risk of developing breast cancer.
- High fat intake increases the risk of developing breast cancer.
- Regular mammography weakly increases the risk of developing breast cancer.
- Eating red meat regularly premenopause moderately increases the risk of developing breast cancer.
- Regular exercise decreases the risk of developing breast cancer (more in premenopause women).
- Breastfeeding weakly decreases the risk of developing breast cancer.

Similarly:

- African American women with breast cancer are more likely to die from it than Caucasians.

Recommendations

- Eliminate/avoid/attenuate risk factors, if possible (please see above and below).
- Self-check breasts once a month, 3–5 days after the menstrual period ended.
- Have a thorough medical checkup once a year.
- Mammograms should be performed every 1–2 years for women over 40.
- Women with a high risk should have annual mammography, annual breast magnetic resonance imaging, and a clinical breast exam every 6–12 months starting as early as age 25 with no upper age limit.
- Regular mammograms significantly reduce the risk of a late-stage breast cancer diagnosis in women 80 years of age and older.

1.5.1.2   Preventive Advice

Chemical

- Forego hormone therapy at menopause, if possible.
- For women at high risk for breast cancer or over the age of 60, certain hormone replacement drugs, such as tamoxifen and raloxifene, have been shown to reduce the risk of breast cancer. Risks and benefits of using these medications should be discussed with physicians.
- Vitamins A, C, and E may decrease the risk of developing breast cancer.
- The correlation between sun exposure and breast cancer prevalence data shows that vitamin D can help prevent breast cancer.

- Calcium and selenium may decrease the risk of developing breast cancer.
- Aspirin may help prevent breast cancer.

Lifestyle

- Breastfeed children and the longer the better.
- Exercise regularly (please see Sect. 2.1).
- Calculate BMI and lose weight, if necessary, by increasing caloric output through exercising and decreasing caloric intake through dieting.
- Do not smoke/stop smoking or chewing tobacco (please see Sect. 2.3).

Nutrition

- Drink alcohol with moderation (please see Sect. 2.4).
- Omega-3 fatty acids in foods may help prevent breast cancer.

1.6   Celiac Disease

1.6.1   Risk Assessment and Prevention of Celiac Disease

1.6.1.1   Risk Assessment

Genetic Markers

- HLA heterodimers, namely, DQ2 (encoded by the DQA1*05 and DQB1*02 alleles) and DQ8 (DQA1*03 and DQB1*0302), are necessary for the development of celiac disease. More than 90 % of patients with celiac disease have these markers (compared to about 40 % in the general population). Please see Table 1.11.
- Many SNPs are linked with an associated risk of developing celiac disease.

  - A large study of 2,000+ celiac disease patients found SNP associations in seven chromosomal regions. Six of these regions harbor genes controlling immune responses, including CCR3, IL-12A, IL-18RAP, RGS1, SH2B3 (rs3184504), and TAGAP.
  - However, some have been disproven. Therefore, one should be cautious not to draw hasty conclusions from genetic test results. For example, please see Table 1.12 for some SNPs associated with celiac disease.

Table 1.11 Blood HLA tests for celiac disease

Test	Sensitivity (%)	Specificity (%)
HLA-DQ2	94	73
HLA-DQ8	12	81

Table 1.12 Analysis of ten celiac disease-associated SNPs reported from a Spanish and a UK study

| SNP | Spanish study | | | | UK genome-wide association study | | | | |
	Allele 1/2	MAF cases	MAF controls	p value	Method	Allele minor/ major	MAF cases	MAF controls	p value
rs12619019	G/C	0.18	0.11	.0015	Imputation INFO=0.90	G/C	0.173	0.162	.33
rs6747096	G/A	0.16	0.29	2.38×10^{-5}	Imputation INFO=0.97	G/A	0.211	0.182	.016
rs11954744	A/T	0.13	0.21	.0016	Imputation INFO=0.93	A/T	0.179	0.164	.19
rs6887645	A/G	0.13	0.21	.0022	Imputation INFO=0.93	A/G	0.180	0.164	.17
rs365836	G/A	0.24	0.33	.0016	Illumina Hap300	G/A	0.256	0.267	.40
rs1048251	T/G	0.53	0.40	3.02×10^{-4}	Imputation INFO=1.03	T/G	0.464	0.444	.21
rs7019234	G/A	0.53	0.40	3.08×10^{-4}	Imputation INFO=1.03	G/A	0.464	0.444	.21
rs459311	T/G	0.52	0.39	1.38×10^{-4}	Imputation INFO=0.99	T/G	0.434	0.434	.21
rs458046	T/A	0.52	0.39	1.35×10^{-4}	Imputation INFO=0.99	T/A	0.435	0.435	.21
rs7040561	T/A	0.15	0.06	6.55×10^{-5}	Imputation INFO=0.77	T/A	0.157	0.141	.12

From: *Gastroenterology* (2008) 134(5–5):1629–1630
SNP imputation was performed using celiac UKGWAS data merged with 2,244,775 high-quality SNPs from 60 CEU founders from the HapMap project
MAF minor allele frequency

Biochemical and Serological Markers

- Serologic testing for celiac disease in children less than 5 years of age may be less reliable than in adults and requires further study.
- Serum antibody tests include the IgA antihuman tissue transglutaminase (TTG) and IgA endomysial antibody immunofluorescence (EMA). They appear to have equivalent diagnostic accuracy (TTG is the specific protein that is identified by the IgA-EMA). Please see Table 1.13 for serologic tests for celiac disease.
- Please see Table 1.11 for blood HLA tests for celiac disease.

Past Medical History

- Timing of the exposure to gluten in childhood is an important risk modifier. People exposed to wheat, barley, or rye within the first 3 months after birth have five times the risk of developing celiac disease relative to those exposed at

Table 1.13 Serologic tests for celiac disease

Antibody type	Substrate or antigen	Test	Sensitivity (%)	Specificity (%)
IgA	Gliadin	ELISA	31–100	85–100
IgG	Gliadin	ELISA	46–100	67–100
IgA	Endomysium	IFA	57–100	95–100
IgA	Reticulin	IFA	29–100	95–100
IgA	Tissue transglutaminase	ELISA	?–100	?–100

From: *Am J Clin Nutr* (1999) 69(3):354–365
Ig immunoglobulin, *ELISA* enzyme-linked immunosorbent assay, *IFA* immunofluorescence assay

4–6 months after birth. Those exposed later than 6 months after birth have only a slightly increased risk relative to those exposed at 4–6 months after birth.
- People with unexplained delayed puberty have an increased risk of developing celiac disease.
- Women with unexplained fetal loss have an increased risk of developing celiac disease.
- Prior depression increases the risk of celiac disease at odds ratio of 2.3.
- People with short stature have an increased risk of developing celiac disease.

Family History

- First-degree relatives have a 1 in 22 chance of developing celiac disease in their lifetimes.
- In second-degree relatives (aunt, uncle, cousin, grandparent), the risk is 1 in 39.

Comorbidities

- Please see Table 1.14 for groups with high prevalence of celiac disease.
- There is a positive correlation between celiac disease and Addison's disease, myasthenia gravis, Raynaud's phenomenon, scleroderma, and systemic lupus erythematosus.
- Dematitis herpetiformis is a risk factor for developing celiac disease.
- People with microscopic colitis have an increased risk of developing celiac disease.
- People with recurrent migraine have an increased risk of developing celiac disease.
- Celiac disease has been associated with sarcoidosis.
- Folic acid deficiency anemia is a risk factor for developing celiac disease.

Similarly:

- Celiac disease is a risk factor for developing pneumococcal infections.

Table 1.14 Groups with high prevalence of celiac disease

Conditions linked with particularly high risk	Conditions linked with higher-than-average risk
Iron deficiency anemia	Type 1 diabetes mellitus
Premature osteoporosis	Autoimmune thyroid disease
Down syndrome	Sjögren syndrome
Unexplained elevations in liver enzymes	Selective IgA deficiency
Primary biliary cirrhosis	Irritable bowel syndrome
Autoimmune hepatitis	Turner's syndrome
	Peripheral neuropathy
	Cerebellar ataxia

From: the American Gastroenterological Association (AGA) Institute

Age/Gender/Ethnicity/Nutrition/Lifestyle

- A meta-analysis indicated that prolonging breastfeeding until the introduction of gluten-containing grains into the diet was associated with a 52 % reduced risk of developing celiac disease in infancy; whether this persists into adulthood is not clear.

Recommendations

- Eliminate/avoid/attenuate risk factors, if possible (please see above and below).
- If any doubt, a small bowel biopsy can rule out celiac disease.
- Pneumococcal vaccine must be taken by adults with celiac disease.

1.6.1.2 Preventive Advice

Chemical

- Check if vitamin and mineral supplements are needed, in particular:
- Calcium
- Folate
- Iron
- Vitamin B12
- Vitamin D
- Vitamin K

Lifestyle

- Breastfeed until the introduction of gluten-containing grains.

Nutrition

• Gluten-free diet (at first avoid also milk and milk products).

1.7   Colorectal Cancer

1.7.1   Risk Assessment and Prevention of Colorectal Cancer (CRC)

1.7.1.1   Risk Assessment

Genetic Markers

• DNA testing of stool samples can be used to screen for CRC.
• Variant rs6983267 on chromosome 8q24 is significantly associated with colorectal cancer. The risk is increased by 20 % for people who have it and it is not modified by other risk factors for CRC.
• The frequency of rs6983267 varies widely among different ethnic groups, from 31 % in ethnic Hawaiians to 85 % in black Americans.
• The analysis of the DNA samples from a polyp can show cancerous characteristics, particularly (1) chromosome instability and gene loss manifested by widespread alterations in chromosome number (aneuploidy); (2) detectable losses at the molecular level of portions of chromosomes 5q, 18q, and 17p; and (3) mutation of the KRAS oncogene. The important genes involved in these chromosome losses are APC (5q), DCC/MADH2/MADH4 (18q), and TP53 (17p).
• Please see Tables 1.15, 1.16, and 1.17 for CRC genetics.

Biochemical and Serological Markers

• Combined CEA and VEGF blood level assay constitutes a useful panel in detecting patients with CRC.
• The combination of plasma TIMP-1 and CEA protein measurements is a potential aid in early detection of CRC and specifically of colon cancer.
• Tests are available to monitor therapy and recurrence risk of CRC. Please see Table 1.18.

Past Medical History

• People with adenomatous polyps have an increased risk of developing CRC.

Table 1.15 Genes responsible for known polyposis and CRC syndromes

Syndrome	Gene	Location	Inheritance	Function	Method of discovery
FAP	*APC*	5q	AD	Inhibition of wnt signaling; ?chromosome segregation	Linkage analysis
HNPCC	*MLH1*	3p	AD	DNA mismatch repair	Linkage analysis
	MSH2	2p	AD	DNA mismatch repair	Linkage analysis
	MSH6	2p	AD	DNA mismatch repair	Candidate gene
	PMS2	7p	AD	DNA mismatch repair	Candidate gene
MAP	*MYH*	1p	AR	Base excision repair	Somatic mutation screening
Peutz–Jeghers	*LKB1*	19p	AD	Serine threonine kinase; ?cell polarity	CGH and linkage analysis
Juvenile polyposis	*SMAD4*	18q	AD	TGF-beta signaling	Candidate linkage analysis
	ALK3	10q	AD	TGF-beta + BMP signaling	Linkage analysis
Cowden's	*PTEN*	10q	AD	Phosphatase, inhibition of AKT signaling	Somatic screening, linkage analysis

AD autosomal dominant, *AR* autosomal recessive, *CGH* comparative genomic hybridization

Table 1.16 Genes associated with a high susceptibility of colorectal cancer

Gene	Syndrome	Hereditary pattern	Predominant cancer
Tumor-suppressor genes			
APC (OMIM)	FAP	Dominant	Colon, intestine, etc.
TP53 (*p53*) (OMIM)	Li–Fraumeni	Dominant	Multiple (including colon)
STK11 (*LKB1*) (OMIM)	PJS	Dominant	Multiple (including intestine)
PTEN (OMIM)	Cowden	Dominant	Multiple (including intestine)
BMPR1A (OMIM)	JPS	Dominant	Gastrointestinal
SMAD4 (*MADH/DPC4*) (OMIM)	JPS	Dominant	Gastrointestinal
Repair/stability genes			
MLH1 (OMIM), *MSH2* (OMIM),*MSH6* (OMIM), *PMS2* (OMIM)	LS	Dominant	Multiple (including colon, uterus, and others)
EPCAM (*TACSTD1*) (OMIM)	LS	Dominant	Multiple (including colon, uterus, and others)
MYH (*MUTYH*) (OMIM)	MYH-associated polyposis	Recessive	

From: the National Cancer Institute
FAP familial adenomatous polyposis, *JPS* juvenile polyposis syndrome, *LS* Lynch syndrome, *OMIM* Online Mendelian Inheritance in Man database, *PJS* Peutz–Jeghers syndrome

Table 1.17 Colorectal cancer susceptibility loci identified through genome-wide association studies

Chromosome	Logarithm of the odds (LOD) score/odds ratio (OR)	p value	Single-nucleotide polymorphism (SNP)	Marker
3q29	LOD = 2.61	.0003		D3S240
4q31.3	LOD = 2.13	.0009		D4S2999
7q31.31	LOD = 3.08	.00008		D7S643
8q23.3	Combined OR = 1.29	1.1×10^{-10}	rs11986063	
8q23.3	$OR_{allelic} = 1.25$, $OR_{het} = 1.27$, $OR_{hom} = 1.43$	3.3×10^{-18}	rs16892766	
	Combined OR = 1.32	1.1×10^{-10}		
8q24	$OR_{allelic} = 1.24$, $OR_{het} = 1.35$, $OR_{hom} = 1.57$	7.0×10^{-11}	rs6983267	
	Combined OR = 0.83	2.1×10^{-14}		
8q24	OR = 1.19	8.6×10^{-26}	rs7014346	
	Combined OR = 1.21	3.0×10^{-13}		
8q24	Combined OR = 1.17	1.2×10^{-10}	rs7837328	
8q24	Combined OR = 1.14	1.5×10^{-7}	rs10808555	
10p14	$OR_{allelic} = 0.89$, $OR_{het} = 0.87$, $OR_{hom} = 0.80$	2.5×10^{-13}	rs10795668	
	Combined OR = 0.91	3.1×10^{-4}		
11q23	OR = 1.11	5.8×10^{-10}	rs3802842	
	Combined OR = 1.21	5.2×10^{-13}		
14q22.2	Combined OR = 1.11	8.1×10^{-10}	rs4444235	
15q13	$OR_{allelic} = 1.23$, $OR_{het} = 1.17$, $OR_{hom} = 1.70$	4.7×10^{-7}	rs4779584	
	Combined OR = 1.19	1.7×10^{-8}		
16q22.1	Combined OR = 0.91	1.2×10^{-8}	rs9929218	
17p13.3[a]	Not available	.0364		D17S1308
18q21	$OR_{allelic} = 0.85$, $OR_{het} = 0.84$, $OR_{hom} = 0.73$	1.7×10^{-6}	rs4939827	
	OR = 1.20	7.8×10^{-28}		
	Combined OR = 0.85	2.2×10^{-11}		
19q13.1	Combined OR = 0.89	2.2×10^{-7}	rs7259371	
19q13.1	Combined OR = 0.87	4.6×10^{-9}	rs10411210	
20p12.3	Combined OR = 1.12	2.0×10^{-10}	rs355527	
20p12.3	Combined OR = 1.12	$2.1\ 10^{-10}$	rs961253	

From: the National Cancer Institute
OR het odds ratio among heterozygotes, *OR hom* odds ratio among homozygotes
[a]Identified in a breast/colon cohort

- Inflammatory bowel disease (ulcerative colitis and Crohn's disease) increases the risk of developing CRC:
  - 5–10 % after 20 years
  - 20 % after 30 years
- Patients with a family or personal history of gynecologic cancer have an increased risk of developing CRC.

Table 1.18 Tests available to select and monitor therapy and recurrence risk of CRC

CA 19-9, serum	Immunochemiluminometric assay	Monitor therapeutic response, detect residual disease, detect recurrence
Carcinoembryonic antigen (CEA)	Immunochemiluminometric assay	
CellSearch circulating tumor cells, colon	Immunomagnetic enrichment of epithelial cells; counting of cells labeled with fluorescent monoclonal antibodies	Predict progression-free and overall survival; monitor treatment response
Dihydropyrimidine Dehydrogenase (DPD) Gene mutation analysis	PCR amplification of target regions followed by hybridization with mutant and wild-type oligonucleotides	Predict toxicity from pyrimidine-based chemotherapeutic agents (5-fluorouracil, capecitabine)
Epidermal growth factor receptor (EGFR), ELISA	Immunoassay	Determine suitability for EGFR-targeted drugs
Epidermal growth factor receptor (EGFR), IHC	Immunohistochemical assay	
FISH, *EGFR*	Fluorescence in situ hybridization	
UGT1A gene Polymorphism (TA repeat)	PCR amplification of promoter region of *UGT1A1*; fluorescent detection	Predict irinotecan toxicity; assist in selecting initial dosage for patients

From: http://www.questdiagnostics.com/testcenter/testguide.action?dc=CF_CRC

Table 1.19 Estimated relative and absolute risk of developing CRC

Family history	Relative risk for CRC	Absolute risk for CRC by age 79 (%)
No family history	1	4
One first-degree relative with CRC	2.3 (95 % CI, 2.0–2.5)	9
More than one first-degree relative with CRC	4.3 (95 % CI, 3.0–6.1)	16
One affected first-degree relative diagnosed with CRC before age 45 years	3.9 (95 % CI, 2.4–6.2)	15
One first-degree relative with colorectal adenoma	2.0 (95 % CI, 1.6–2.6)	8

Family History

- 25 % of patients with CRC have a positive family history. Please see Table 1.19.
- Familial adenomatous polyposis (FAP) increases the risk of developing CRC beginning during the teenage years. If untreated, the risk of developing colon cancer is nearly 100 %, usually before age 40.
- The MYH-associated polyposis (MAP) risk is similar to FAP's.
- Gardner's syndrome (a variant of FAP) increases the risk of developing CRC.

- Lynch syndrome increases the risk of developing CRC. Also called hereditary nonpolyposis colorectal cancer (HNPCC), it has the following characteristics:
  - It represents 3 % of all colorectal cancers.
  - Cancer risk is 70 % by age 65.
  - In about 70 % of families, there is mutation in one of four genes.
- Please see Table 1.19 for family history and estimated relative and absolute risk of developing CRC.

Comorbidities

- Type 2 diabetes increases the risk of developing CRC by 30–40 %.
- Overweight and obesity increase the risk of developing CRC.
- Peutz–Jeghers syndrome increases the risk of developing CRC.
- Barrett's esophagus increases the risk of developing CRC.
- Human immunodeficiency virus infection increases the risk of developing CRC.
- Acromegaly increases the risk of developing CRC.
- Inflammatory bowel disease increases the risk of developing CRC.
- Stomach cancer (HDGC) increases the risk of developing HNPCC.

Age/Gender/Ethnicity/Nutrition/Lifestyle

- CRC affects an equal number of men and women.
- 90 % of all CRC occur after age 50.
- Ashkenazi Jews (I 1307 K APC mutation) have a lifetime CRC risk of 9–15 %. This risk elevation is similar to that of individuals in the familial risk category.
- African Americans have a higher risk of developing CRC.
- Smoking significantly increases the risk for colon polyps and colon cancer.
- Drinking alcohol, especially beer, increases the risk of developing polyps and CRC.
- Red meat (beef, pork, lamb) and processed meat (hot dogs, bacon, cold cuts) increase the risk of developing CRC.
- Sedentarity increases the risk of developing polyps and CRC and physical activity decreases the risk of developing CRC.
- The incidence of CRC is highest in industrialized nations and lowest in Asia, Africa, and South America.
- A diet high in fruits and vegetables decreases the risk of developing CRC.

Recommendations

- Eliminate/avoid/attenuate risk factors, if possible (please see above and below).
- Men and women over 50 should be screened according to the guidelines included in Tables 1.20 and 1.21:

Table 1.20 Tests that detect adenomatous polyps and cancer

Test	Interval	Key issues for informed decisions
Flexible sigmoidoscopy (FSIG) with insertion to 40 cm or to splenic flexure	Every 5 years	Complete or partial bowel prep is required
		Sedation usually is not used, so there may be some discomfort during the procedure
		The protective effect of sigmoidoscopy is primarily limited to the portion of the colon examined
		Patients should understand that positive findings on sigmoidoscopy usually result in a referral for colonoscopy
Colonoscopy	Every 10 years	Complete bowel prep is required
		Conscious sedation is used in most centers; patients will miss a day of work and will need a chaperone for transportation from the facility
		Risks include perforation and bleeding, which are rare but potentially serious; most of the risk is associated with polypectomy
Double contrast barium enema (DCBE)	Every 5 years	Complete bowel prep is required
		If patients have one or more polyps ≥6 mm, colonoscopy will be recommended; follow-up colonoscopy will require complete bowel prep
		Risks of DCBE are low; rare cases of perforation have been reported
Computed tomographic colonography (CTC)	Every 5 years	Complete bowel prep is required
		If patients have one or more polyps ≥6 mm, colonoscopy will be recommended; if same-day colonoscopy is not available, a second complete bowel prep will be required before colonoscopy
		Risks of CTC are low; rare cases of perforation have been reported
		Extracolonic abnormalities may be identified on CTC that could require further evaluation

From: American College of Gastroenterology

1.7.1.2 Preventive Advice

Chemical

- Regular aspirin use may reduce the risk of developing polyps and CRC but it increases the risk of gastrointestinal bleeding.
- For women in post menopause, hormone therapy may reduce the risk of CRC. However, it also increases the risk of breast cancer, dementia, heart disease, stroke, and blood clots.
- HMG-CoA reductase inhibitors (statins) may protect against CRC.
- Calcium protects against CRC.
- Vitamin D, which aids in the absorption of calcium, also appears to help reduce the risk of CRC.

Table 1.21 Tests that primarily detect CRC

Test	Interval	Key issues for informed decisions
Guaiac-based fecal occult blood test (gFOBT) with high sensitivity for cancer	Annual	Depending on manufacturer's recommendations, 2 to 3 stool samples collected at home are needed to complete testing; a single sample of stool gathered during a digital exam in the clinical setting is not an acceptable stool test and should not be done
Fecal immunochemical test (FIT) with high sensitivity for cancer	Annual	Positive tests are associated with an increased risk of colon cancer and advanced neoplasia; colonoscopy should be recommended if the test results are positive
		If the test is negative, it should be repeated annually
		Patients should understand that one-time testing is likely to be ineffective
Stool DNA (sDNA) with high sensitivity for cancer	Interval uncertain	An adequate stool sample must be obtained and packaged with appropriate preservative agents for shipping to the laboratory
		The unit cost of the currently available test is significantly higher than other forms of stool testing
		If the test is positive, colonoscopy will be recommended
		If the test is negative, the appropriate interval for a repeat test is uncertain

From: American College of Gastroenterology

- Antioxidants such as selenium, beta-carotene, and lutein help prevent CRC.
- Folic acid is useful in protecting against CRC.

Lifestyle

- Know about CRC (please see Sect. 2.9).
- Exercise regularly (please see Sect. 2.1).
- Do not smoke/quit smoking or chewing tobacco (please see Sect. 2.3).
- Control body weight.
- Sun exposure before 10 am and after 3 pm protects against CRC (by metabolizing calcium).
- Action plans may vary for people at high risk for CRC, for example:

  – If at risk for familial adenomatous polyposis (FAP) because of a family history of the disease, consider having genetic counseling.
  – If diagnosed with FAP, regular colonoscopy tests should be done, starting in early teens, and other options discussed. Removing the entire colon may be one.
  – People at risk of Lynch syndrome should begin having regular colonoscopies around age 20.
  – In case of genetic cancer syndrome, make sure family members are tested.

Nutrition

- Green tea helps prevent CRC.
- Fiber protects against CRC. It can be found in whole-grain cereals and breads, prunes, berries, kidney beans, and brown rice.
- Plenty of fruits and vegetables should be part of the daily diet. The American Cancer Society recommends eating at least five servings of fruits and vegetables every day (please also see Sect. 2.5).
- Fat intake should be limited to no more than 10 % of daily calorie intake.
- Consumption of red and processed meat should be limited.
- Alcohol consumption should be moderate (please see Sect. 2.4).

1.8 Crohn's Disease

1.8.1 Risk Assessment and Prevention of Crohn's Disease

1.8.1.1 Risk Assessment

Genetic Markers

- DNA variations on chromosomes 1 and 3 show evidence of genes that cause Crohn's disease (specifically in Ashkenazi families).
- Genetic abnormalities on chromosomes 13, 2, and 19 appear to increase the risk of developing Crohn's disease in Jewish and non-Jewish families.
- People with an abnormal mutation or alteration in a gene NOD2/CARD 15 have an increased risk of developing Crohn's disease.
- The gene ATG16L1 is implicated in Crohn's disease.
- Over 30 genes have been associated with Crohn's disease such as TNF, DLG5, NCF4 etc. For some example please see Table 1.22.

Biochemical and Serological Markers

- Several serological markers such as ASCA, ACMA, ALCA, ACCA, ASigmaMA, OmpC, CBir1, and 12 others have been associated with an increased risk of developing Crohn's disease. Please see Table 1.23.

- "A number of neutrophil derived proteins present in stools have been studied, including faecal lactoferrin, lysozyme, elastase, myeloperoxidase, and calprotectin. Calprotectin, a 36 kDa calcium and zinc binding protein, is probably the most promising marker. In contrast with other neutrophil markers, calprotectin represents 60 % of cytosolic proteins in granulocytes. The presence of calprotectin in faeces can therefore be seen as directly proportional to neutrophil migration to

Table 1.22 Summary of the GWA study and replication studies

Rank	Number of SNPs	Chr	RS number	GWA MAF iCD	GWA MAF CTL	GWA p value	Replication cohort 1 T	Replication cohort 1 U	Replication cohort 2 MAF iCD	Replication cohort 2 MAF CTL	Combined replication OR	Combined replication p value	Gene
1	8	16	rs2076756	0.358	0.244	7.01×10^{-14}	P.T.	P.T.	P.T.	P.T.	P.T.	P.T.	CARD15
2	13	1	rs7517847	0.295	0.403	3.06×10^{-12}	P.T.	P.T.	P.T.	P.T.	P.T.	P.T.	IL-23R
3	3	2	rs2241880	0.364	0.453	6.38×10^{-8}	220	306	0.353	0.478	0.68	4.1×10^{-8}	ATG16L1
4	1	4	rs16853571	0.038	0.077	7.68×10^{-7}	39	75	0.057	0.047	0.69	0.0084	PHOX2B
5	1	12	rs886898	0.156	0.102	1.93×10^{-6}	121	136	N.D.	N.D.	N.D.	N.D.	–
6	2	1	rs2343331	0.279	0.212	2.49×10^{-6}	Failed	Failed	N.D.	N.D.	N.D.	N.D.	–
7	1	18	rs937815	0.054	0.094	3.25×10^{-6}	96	99	N.D.	N.D.	N.D.	N.D.	–
8	1	3	rs6439924	0.218	0.160	6.00×10^{-6}	166	140	N.D.	N.D.	N.D.	N.D.	–
9	1	10	rs224136	0.134	0.191	7.90×10^{-6}	94	149	0.140	0.230	0.60	2.9×10^{-7}	Intergenic
10	1	9	rs10821091	0.399	0.332	1.44×10^{-5}	274	252	N.D.	N.D.	N.D.	N.D.	–
11	1	14	rs1188157	0.487	0.417	1.58×10^{-5}	254	240	N.D.	N.D.	N.D.	N.D.	–
12	1	1	rs2819130	0.177	0.126	2.10×10^{-5}	130	144	N.D.	N.D.	N.D.	N.D.	–
13	1	11	rs2712800	0.373	0.441	2.38×10^{-5}	242	222	N.D.	N.D.	N.D.	N.D.	–

(continued)

Table 1.22 (continued)

Rank	Chr	Number of SNPs	RS number	GWA			Replication cohort 1		Replication cohort 2		Combined replication		Gene
				MAF iCD	MAF CTL	p value	T	U	MAF iCD	MAF CTL	OR	p value	
14	22	1	**rs4821544**	0.397	0.333	2.89×10^{-5}	267	221	0.374	0.339	1.19	0.0090	*NCF4*
15	2	1	**rs6733000**	0.081	0.124	3.03×10^{-5}	81	77	N.D.	N.D.	N.D.	N.D.	–
16	2	1	**rs7603516**	0.064	0.102	3.10×10^{-5}	73	62	N.D.	N.D.	N.D.	N.D.	–
17	16	1	**rs8050910**	0.388	0.458	3.28×10^{-5}	221	271	0.400	0.430	0.84	0.0085	*FAM92B*
18	1	2	**rs2490271**	0.206	0.152	3.44×10^{-5}	175	166	N.D.	N.D.	N.D.	N.D.	–
19	20	1	**rs4810663**	0.236	0.180	3.45×10^{-5}	182	178	N.D.	N.D.	N.D.	N.D.	–
20	8	1	**rs10505007**	0.400	0.332	3.78×10^{-5}	221	248	N.D.	N.D.	N.D.	N.D.	–
21	8	1	**rs2044999**	0.330	0.395	3.84×10^{-5}	NT	NT	N.D.	N.D.	N.D.	N.D.	–
22	9	1	**rs4878061**	0.418	0.485	4.64×10^{-5}	NT	NT	N.D.	N.D.	N.D.	N.D.	–
23	13	1	**rs11617463**	0.044	0.077	4.85×10^{-5}	59	80	Failed	Failed	N.D.	N.D.	–

From: *Nat Genet* (2007) 39:596–604. doi:10.1038/ng2032

The GWA study was performed in 946 individuals with ileal Crohn's disease and 977 controls. The replication studies were performed in 530 trios with ileal Crohn's disease (replication cohort 1) and 350 cases with ileal Crohn's disease and 207 controls (replication cohort 2). The 23 top-ranked regions ($p < 5 \times 10^{-5}$) in the GWA analysis that we included in the replication study are listed in order of significance. The number of SNPs falling below this threshold within each region is indicated. *p* values are two tailed for the GWA results and one tailed for the combined replication study. SNPs in boldface are those with significant evidence of replication (replication cohort 1)

OR odds ratio

Table 1.23 Diagnostic accuracy of individual serological markers and their combinations in differential diagnosis of CD and UC

Diagnosis	Antibody	Sensitivity (%)	Specificity (%)	PPV	NPV
CD	ASCA +	37–72	82–100	87–95	36–68
	pANCA −	52	91	85	65
	ACCA	9–21	84–97	78–87	24–52
	ALCA	15–26	92–96	78–90	25–53
	AMCA	12–28	82–97	65–92	25–52
	Anti-C	10–25	90–98	87–88	29–39
	Anti-L	18–26	93–97	90–91	30–40
	Anti-OmpC	20–55	81–88	83	25
	Anti-I2	42	76	NR	NR
	PAB	22–46	77–100	69–100	48–75
	ASCA+/pANCA−	46–64	92–99	86–97	44–82
	PAB+/ANCA−	22–42	98–100	87–100	48–74
	PAB+/ASCA+/pANCA−	16–34	97–100	100	66–72
UC	pANCA	50–71	75–98	74–95	49–84
	pANCA+/ASCA−	42–58	81–100	93–100	43
	GAB	12[a]–46	98	75–93	70–74
	pANCA or GAB+/PAB−	82	98	96	89

From: *Biochemia Medica* (2013);23(1):28–42. http://dx.doi.org/10.11613/BM.2013.006
PPV positive predictive value, *NPV* negative predictive value, *ASCA* Anti-Saccharomyces cerevisiae antibodies, *pANCA* anti-neutrophil cytoplasmic antibodies, *ACCA* antichitobioside carbohydrate antibodies, *ALCA* antilaminaribioside carbohydrate antibodies, *AMCA* anti-mannobioside carbohydrate antibodes, *Anti-C* anti-chitin antibodies, *Anti-L* anti-laminarin antibodies, *Anti-OmpC* antibody to outer membrane porin C, *Anti-I2* antibody to *Pseudomonas fluorescens* – associated sequence I2, *PAB* antibodies against exocrine pancreas, *GAB* antibodies to goblet cells, *NR* not reported
[a]In pediatric population

the gastrointestinal tract. Although calprotectin is a very sensitive marker for detection of inflammation in the gastrointestinal tract, it is not a specific marker and increased levels are found in neoplasia, IBD, infections, and polyps. Five faecal calprotectin is a very stable marker (stable for more than 1 week at room temperature) and is resistant to degradation, which makes it attractive." (From: Gut (2006) 55(3):426–431)

Family History

- A close relative, such as a parent, sibling, or child, with the disease increases the risk of developing Crohn's disease (up to one in five people with Crohn's disease has a family member with the disease).

Comorbidities

- Please see Table 1.24, for secondary health problems in patients with inflammatory bowel disease.

Table 1.24 Putting comorbidity into context: secondary health problems in patients with inflammatory bowel disease

Extraintestinal manifestations	Adverse effects of treatments	Comorbidities	Direct consequences of the disease
Peripheral and axial arthritis	Steroids: cataracts, glaucoma, mood changes, osteoporosis, etc.	Cardiovascular	Abdominal and retroperitoneal scarring: hydronephrosis, intestinal obstruction, female infecundity, etc.
Erythema nodosum, pyoderma gangrenosum, oral aphthae	Immunosuppressors: infections, neoplasia, liver toxicity, myelosuppression, etc.	Hepatic, biliary, pancreatic, digestive	Consequences of intestinal resection: malabsorption, short bowel syndrome, oxalate nephrolithiasis
Uveitis, episcleritis, blepharitis	Biologics: infections, neoplasia, demyelinizing disease, infusion	Metabolic: obesity	Persistent inflammation: osteoporosis, amyloidosis
Primary sclerosing cholangitis	Reactions, drug-induced lupus	Neuropsychiatric	

From: *World J Gastroenterol* (2011) 17(22):2723–2733

Age/Gender/Ethnicity/Nutrition/Lifestyle

- Crohn's disease is more frequent in women.
- Women taking oral contraceptives have twice the risk of developing Crohn's disease, As those who don't.
- Hormone replacement therapy increases the risk of developing Crohn's disease.
- Young age increases the risk of developing Crohn's disease. Most people who have Crohn's disease are diagnosed before they reach 30 years old.
- Crohn's disease presents two peaks: between 15 and 40 years of age and between 50 and 80 years of age.
- Left-handed individuals have twice the risk of right-handed persons of developing Crohn's disease.
- Eastern Europeans of Jewish descent (Ashkenazi) have an increased risk of developing Crohn's disease.
- Present or past smoking increases the risk of developing Crohn's disease.
- Hypersensitivity to cow's milk and consumption of a low-fiber diet, refined sugar, and fat food increase the risk of developing Crohn's disease.
- There is some evidence of NSAID-induced Crohn's disease in the small and large bowel.
- Appendectomy in adulthood increases the risk of developing Crohn's disease, but it decreases it if it was performed before 20 years of age.

- Living in an urban area or in an industrialized country increases the risk of developing Crohn's disease.
- Living in northern climates also seems to increase the risk of developing Crohn's disease.
- Dysbiosis due to infection or antibiotic use appears to be a risk factor for developing Crohn's disease.
- Stress can be a contributing factor in Crohn's disease.
- Breastfeeding protects against Crohn's disease.

Similarly:

- Obese people are more likely to have an active disease and require more hospitalizations.

Recommendations

- Eliminate/avoid/attenuate risk factors, if possible (please see above and below).

1.8.1.2 Preventive Advice

Chemical

- Consider multivitamins.
- Add probiotics to the diet.
- Add fish oil to the diet.

Lifestyle

- Breastfeed.
- Control weight. Lose some, if necessary, by decreasing caloric input (through dieting) and increasing caloric output (through exercising).
- Get regular exercise (please see Sect. 2.1).
- Do not smoke/quit smoking or chewing tobacco (please see Sect. 2.3).
- Reduce stress (please see Sect. 2.2).
- Get enough sleep (please see Sect. 2.2).
- Avoid OCP, HRT, and NSAIDs, if possible.
- Avoid urban areas, if possible.
- Avoid cold climates, if possible.

Nutrition

- Limit refined sugar intake.
- Limit dairy products.

- Eat low-fat foods (foods to avoid include butter, margarine, cream sauces, and fried foods). The Stanford Health Improvement Program recommends the Mediterranean diet.
- Eat the recommended daily amount of fruits and vegetables (please see Sect. 2.5).
- Eat small meals.
- Have a sufficient fiber intake. For every 1,000 cal try to have at least 14 g of fiber.
- Drink plenty of fluids daily (water is best).

1.9   Deep Venous Thrombosis

1.9.1   Risk Assessment and Prevention of Deep Venous Thrombosis (DVT)

1.9.1.1   Risk Assessment

Genetic Markers

- There is a positive association between DVT and 3 common variants of CYP4V2, a cytochrome p450 gene, SERPINC1, and GP6.
- Factor V mutation (Arg 506rGln), protein C and S, and antithrombin III gene defects are risk factors for developing DVT.
- Please see Tables 1.25 and 1.26 for common variant associations results and nonsynonymous, SNP-variants in anticoagulant genes with likely deleterious effect on the encoded proteins.

Biochemical and Serological Markers

- The presence of the lupus anticoagulant increases the risk of developing DVT.
- Protein C deficiency increases the risk of developing DVT.
- The presence of activated protein C resistance increases the risk of developing DVT.
- Antiphospholipid antibodies increase the risk of developing DVT.
- Factor V Leiden increases the risk of developing DVT.
- Prothrombin G20210A increases the risk of developing DVT.
- Protein S deficiency increases the risk of developing DVT.
- Antithrombin III deficiency is a risk factor for developing DVT.
- Dysfibrinogenemia increases the risk of developing DVT.
- ABO blood group increases the risk of developing DVT.
- Hypercholesterolemia increases the risk of developing DVT.
- Factor II is a risk factor for developing DVT.

Table 1.25 Nonsynonymous single-nucleotide variants in anticoagulant genes

Gene	Chromosome	Coordinate	Substitution	Transcript ID	Protein change	dbSNP129	1,000 genomes CEU population, allele frequency	SIFT[a]	Polyphen 2[b]	Allele cases	Allele controls
PROC	**chr2**	127895370	C>T	NM_000312	p.R38W	**Novel**	Not present	Dam	Prd	2	0
		127902716	C>A		p.H370Q	**Novel**	Not present	Ben	Ben	1	0
SERPINC1	**chr1**	172150549	G>A	NM_000488	p.P58L	**Novel**	Not present	Dam	Pod	1	0
PROZ	**chr13**	112861006	C>G	NM_003891	p.L11V	**Novel**	Not present	Ben	Ben	3	0
		112874101	G>A		p.R295H	**rs3024772**	Not present	Ben	Prd	2	2

From: BMC Med Genomic (2012) 5:7. doi:10.1186/1755-8794-5-7

[a]SIFT-based annotation results. Dam indicates that the mutation is predicted to affect protein function (i.e., "damaging"), and Ben indicates that the mutation is predicted to be tolerated (i.e., "benign")

[b]Polyphen 2-based annotation results. Prd indicates that the mutation is predicted to be "probably damaging," Pod indicates that the mutation is predicted to be "possibly damaging," and Ben indicates that the mutation is predicted to be "benign"

Table 1.26 Common variant association results

Variant information						Discovery			Replication stages 1 and 2 (combined)						
Location	Substitution	Gene	Functional annotation	Protein	dbSNP129	Alleles cases	Alleles controls	$p =$	Effective sample size cases	MAF cases, % (n)	Effective sample size controls	MAF controls, % (n)	$p =$	OR	95 % CI
chr4:155727040	T>C	FGA	Exon missense	p.T331A	rs6050	10	4	0.004	709	32 (453)	702	22 (312)	1.9×10^{-5}	1.45	1.22–1.72
chr16:80474413	A>G	PLCG2	Exon missense	p.H244R	rs11548656	4	0	0.013	711	6 (88)	705	6 (83)	0.73	1.05	0.77–1.43
chr4:122837138	T>C	ANXA5	Intron	Na	rs2306416	4	0	0.013	139	15 (41)	138	15 (42)	0.97	0.96	0.60–1.54
chr8:42164111	G>A	PLAT	Exon synonymous	Na	rs1058720	11	3	0.002	139	47 (131)	139	44 (124)	0.61	1.10	0.79–1.54
chr11:47311481	T>C	MYBPC3	Intron	Na	rs11570115	5	0	0.004	137	11 (30)	139	9 (26)	0.63	1.19	0.68–2.07

From: *BMC Med Genomic* (2012) 5:7. doi:10.1186/1755-8794-5-7

MAF minor allele frequency, *OR* odds ratio, *Na* not applicable (the variant does not cause protein sequence changes), *CI* confidence interval

- Hyperfibrinogenemia increases the risk of developing DVT.
- Raised plasma levels of factor VIII increase the risk of developing DVT.
- Raised plasma levels of homocysteine increase the risk of developing DVT.
- Thrombocythemia increases the risk of developing DVT.

Past Medical History

- Prior history of DVT or pulmonary embolism increases the risk of developing DVT.
- Recent surgery, particularly on the knees, hips, or pelvis, increases the risk of developing DVT.
- Trauma to the vessels increases the risk of developing DVT.
- Birth control pills or hormone replacement therapy increases the risk of developing DVT.
- A pacemaker or a thin, flexible tube (catheter) in a vein increases the risk of developing DVT.

Family History

- For people with no environmental or genetic risk factors, having a first-degree relative (parent or sibling) with DVT increases the odds of having a first episode of DVT by 2.5-folds. This is about the same as the increase in odds (2.3 times) caused by genetic risk factors in people with no family history or environmental risk factors.
- Inheriting a blood clotting disease increases the risk of developing DVT.

Comorbidities

- Polycythemia vera increases the risk of developing DVT.
- Cancers of the brain, ovary, pancreas, colon, stomach, lung, and kidney have the highest risk of DVT.
- Liver cancer can cause DVT.
- Lymphomas and leukemia are likely to lead to DVT.
- Heart failure increases the risk of developing DVT.
- Inflammatory bowel disease such as ulcerative colitis increases the risk of developing DVT.
- Nephrotic syndrome increases the risk of developing DVT.
- Varicose veins increase the risk of developing DVT.
- Admission to an intensive care unit increases the risk of developing DVT.
- Injury or surgery increases the risk of developing DVT.
- Obesity increases the risk of developing DVT.
- Cancer treatment increases the risk of developing DVT.

Age/Gender/Ethnicity/Nutrition/Lifestyle

- Overall, DVT is equally common in women and men.
- The risk of DVT doubles for each 10-year increase in age after 50.
- Women during their childbearing years have a higher risk of developing DVT than men.
- After age 50, men have a risk about 20 % higher than women.
- Unique factors that can put women at risk include:

  - Oral contraceptives that contain estrogen and progestin, which increase a woman's risk of blood clot two to eight times. Because they contain more estrogen, contraceptive patches may carry an even greater risk. Progestin-only contraceptives do not appear to increase risk.
  - Hormone replacement therapy, which increases a woman's risk of DVT by two to four times.
  - Pregnancy and the first few months after the baby is born, which increase the risk of DVT more than fourfold.

- Women who have more than one DVT risk factor, for example, obese women who take oral contraceptives, increase their normal risk by tenfold.
- African Americans are at the greatest risk of developing DVT with a 30 % higher risk than whites.
- People of Asian or Native American backgrounds have a much lower risk of developing DVT, 70 % less than whites.
- Taller men have an increased risk of developing DVT. Taller women do not appear to have an increased risk.
- Overweight increases the pressure in veins of the pelvis and legs, which increases the risk of DVT. Women who are obese (BMI over 30) have two to three times the normal risk of developing DVT.
- Smoking increases the risk of developing DVT.
- Sitting for long periods of time, such as when driving or flying, increases the risk of developing DVT.
- Prolonged bed rest (hospital stay, paralysis) increases the risk of developing DVT.
- Certain medications increase the risk of developing DVT such as erythropoietin, tamoxifen, and thalidomide.

Recommendations

- Eliminate/avoid/attenuate risk factors, if possible (please see above and below).

1.9.1.2 Preventive Advice

Chemical

- N-Acetylcysteine has anticoagulant and platelet-inhibiting properties.
- Vitamin E may reduce the risk of blood clots in women.

- People having surgery, such as orthopedic operations, are usually given blood thinners while in the hospital.

Similarly:

- For people on anticoagulants, watch how much vitamin K is eaten. It can be found in green leafy vegetables and canola and soybean oils and can interfere with warfarin, for example.
- Check regularly to see if anticoagulant treatments need to be adjusted or modified.

Lifestyle

- Get regular exercise (please see Sect. 2.1).
- Exercise calf muscles if sitting for a long time. Whenever possible, get up and walk around. If it is impossible, try raising and lowering heels while keeping the toes on the floor and then raising the toes while heels are on the floor.
- Do not smoke/quit smoking or chewing tobacco (please see Sect. 2.3).
- If necessary, lose weight by increasing caloric output through exercising and decreasing caloric intake through dieting.
- Control blood pressure.
- Wear compression stockings when traveling for long periods of time or during the day, if necessary.
- Do not stay in bed too long when hospitalized and if possible.
- Do not sit too long (e.g., when traveling or in front of a computer).

Nutrition

- Chamomile herb has moderate effects on blood clots and platelet aggregation.
- Cranberry juice, sauce, or cranberry supplements help thin the blood.
- EGCG, the extract from green tea, may prevent platelet aggregation almost as potently as aspirin.
- Garlic has mild antiplatelet activity along with the ability to break down fibrin.
- Nettle herb has antiplatelet activity.

1.10 Diabetes Mellitus (Type 2)

1.10.1 Risk Assessment and Prevention of Type 2 Diabetes Mellitus (DM)

1.10.1.1 Risk Assessment

Genetic Markers

- As of 2011, more than 36 genes had been found that contribute to the risk of type 2 diabetes. They only account for 10 % of the total genetic component of the disease.

- The genetic markers for type 2 diabetes mellitus are many as shown in the table below:

Authors	Outcome	Number of genetic markers	AUC (clinical risk score)	AUC (clinical risk score and genetic markers)	Significant improvement of AUC with genetic markers[a]	Significant improvement of NRI or IDI with genetic markers[b]
Van Hoek et al.	Incident T2D	18	0.66	0.68	Yes	N/A
Lango et al.	Prevalent T2D	18	0.78	0.80	Yes	N/A
Lyssenko et al.	Incident T2D	16	0.74[c]	0.75	Yes	Yes
Meigs et al.	Incident T2D	18	0.900[c]	0.901	No	No
Lin et al.	Prevalent T2D	15	0.86[c]	0.87	Yes	Yes
Sparso et al.	Prevalent T2D	19	0.92	0.93	N/A	N/A
Schulze et al.	Incident T2D	20	0.8626	0.8628	No	No
Cornelis et al.	Incident T2D	10	0.78	0.79	Yes	N/A
Talmud et al.[d]	Incident T2D	20	0.72[c]	0.73	Yes	No
Talmud et al.[d]	Incident T2D	20	0.78[c]	0.78	No	No
Wang et al.[d]	Prevalent T2D	19	0.727[c]	0.730	N/A	N/A
Wang et al.[d]	Prevalent T2D	19	0.772[c]	0.772	N/A	N/A
Qi et al.	Prevalent T2D	17	0.77[c]	0.79	Yes	N/A
de Miguel-Yanes et al.[d]	Incident T2D (in people <50 years)	40	0.908	0.911	No	Yes
de Miguel-Yanes et al.[d]	Incident T2D (in people ≥50 years)	40	0.883	0.884	No	No

AUC area under the receiver operating characteristic curve, *IDI* integrated discrimination improvement, *N/A* not applicable (data not available), *NRI* net reclassification index, *T2D* type 2 diabetes
[a]Improvement of model discrimination or reclassification was considered statistically significant if $p < 0.05$
[b]NRI was statistically significant ($p < 0.05$)
[c]Risk model included family or parental history of diabetes
[d]These studies analyzed two different classical risk scores with increasing complexity reflected by differences in AUC or two different outcomes and are therefore listed twice

Biochemical and Serological Markers

- Tumor necrosis factor-alpha (TNF-α), interleukin-6 (IL-6), and high-sensitivity C-reactive protein (hs-CRP) are significantly related to an increased risk of clinical DM. CRP appears to be a more consistent predictor of increased risk. These associations are independent of the traditional risk factors such as obesity and elevated levels of glucose and insulin.
- HDL <35 mg/dL increases the risk of developing DM.
- TG >250 mg/dL increases the risk of developing DM.
- IFG (impaired fasting glucose) or IGT (impaired glucose tolerance) increases the risk of developing DM.
- For recommended screening tests, please see Table 1.27.

Table 1.27 Tests used in diabetes diagnosis and management

Test name	Primary clinical use and differentiating factors
Glucose, plasma	Diagnosis based on FPG
Glucose tolerance test, 2 specimens (75 g)	Diagnosis based on fasting and 2 h (post 75 g glucose loading) specimens (2 h OGTT)
Glucose tolerance test, gestational, 4 specimens (100 g)	Diagnosis of gestational diabetes
GlycoMark®	Management; measures PPG excursions; may help differentiate contributions of FPG and PPG to hyperglycemia in patients with moderately or well-controlled HbA1c levels
Hemoglobin A1c	Diagnosis and management; determines long-term average blood glucose, expressed as a percentage
Hemoglobin A1c with eAG	Management; determines long-term average blood glucose; expressed in percent HbA1c and conventional blood glucose units for more convenient comparison to SMBG values
Hemoglobin A1c with eAG with reflex to GlycoMark	Management; determines long-term average blood glucose levels, expressed in percent HbA1c and conventional blood glucose units. Measures PPG excursions; may help differentiate contributions of FPG and PPG to hyperglycemia in patients with moderately or well-controlled HbA1c levels
Hemoglobin A1c with reflex to GlycoMark	Management; determines long-term average blood glucose levels, expressed as a percentage. Measures PPG excursions; may help differentiate contributions of FPG and PPG to hyperglycemia in patients with moderately or well-controlled HbA1c levels
Self-monitoring of blood glucose (SMBG)	Management; determines response to insulin therapy on a daily basis

From: https://www.questdiagnostics.com/testcenter/testguide.action?dc=TG_Diabetes

Past Medical History

- Prediabetes often progresses to type 2 diabetes.
- Gestational diabetes increases the risk of developing type 2 diabetes later in life.
- Giving birth to a baby weighing more than 9 lb (4.1 kg) increases the risk of developing type 2 diabetes (macrosomia).
- History of vascular diseases increases the risk of developing DM.
- Insulin resistance disease or condition increases the risk of developing DM (e.g., polycystic ovary syndrome).
- Some medications such as glucocorticoids, thiazides, beta-adrenergic agonists, and alpha interferon increase the risk of developing DM.

Family History

- A person with a family history of DM is two to four times as likely to develop the disease as someone without a family history.

- Versus people in the average risk class, independently of other risk factors, the odds of having diabetes for people in the moderate and high familial risk categories are, respectively, 2.3 and 5.5 times higher.

Comorbidities

The following diseases and conditions increase the risk of developing DM:

- Acromegaly, Cushing's syndrome, hyperthyroidism, pheochromocytoma, certain cancers such as glucagonoma, and testosterone deficiency.
- High blood pressure ($\geq$140/90 mmHg) increases the risk of developing DM.
- Metabolic syndrome increases the risk of developing DM.
- Acanthosis nigricans is a risk factor for developing DM.
- Polycystic ovarian syndrome is a risk factor for developing DM.

Similarly:

- People with DM have an increased risk of developing cardiovascular disorders, including coronary artery diseases and stroke.
- People with DM have an increased risk of developing depression.
- People with DM have an increased risk of developing obstructive sleep apnea.
- People with DM have an increased risk of developing nonalcoholic fatty liver disease.
- People with DM have an increased risk of developing cancer (pancreas, colorectum, breast, bladder, endometrium, liver).
- People with DM have an increased risk of developing adult-onset blindness.
- People with DM have an increased risk of developing fractures.
- People with DM have an increased risk of developing hypertension.
- People with DM have an increased risk of developing renal diseases.
- People with DM have an increased risk of developing hypoglycemia.
- People with DM have an increased risk of developing peripheral vascular disease.
- People with DM have an increased risk of developing dyslipidemia.
- People with DM have an increased risk of being amputated.

Age/Gender/Ethnicity/Nutrition/Lifestyle

- The risk of developing type 2 diabetes increases with age, especially after 45. However, the prevalence of type 2 diabetes is currently also increasing dramatically among children, adolescents, and younger adults.
- Blacks, Hispanics, American Indians, and Asian Americans are more likely to develop type 2 diabetes than Caucasians.
- Being overweight is a primary risk factor for type 2 diabetes. Fatty tissue increases the resistance to insulin.
- If fat is stored primarily in the abdominal area, the risk of developing type 2 diabetes is greater.
- Inactivity increases the risk of developing DM.
- Smoking 16 to 25 cigarettes a day increases the risk of developing DM to 3 times that of a non-smoker.

Recommendations

- Eliminate/avoid/attenuate risk factors, if possible (please see above and below).
- Everyone over 45 should have a glucose test at least every 3 years. Regular testing of blood sugar levels should begin at a younger age and be performed more often if there is a higher risk for diabetes.

1.10.1.2   Preventive Advice

Chemical

- Metformin decreases the risk of developing DM.
- Niacinamide is believed to be effective for DM and also for delaying the need for insulin.
- Vitamin C may help to decrease the risk of developing DM.
- Vitamin D may help to decrease the risk of developing DM.
- Vitamin E may help to decrease the risk of developing DM.
- Calcium may help to decrease the risk of developing DM.

Lifestyle

- Know about diabetes (please see Sect. 2.8).
- Exercise regularly (please see Sect. 2.1).
- Lose weight, if necessary, by increasing caloric output (exercising) and decreasing caloric intake (dieting).
- Reduce stress (please see Sect. 2.2).
- Do not smoke/stop smoking or chewing tobacco (please see Sect. 2.3).

Nutrition

- Reduce glucose intake from unnecessary sources (sweets, desserts, sodas, etc.).
- Choose foods low in fat and calories.
- Eat chemical-free food.
- Be suspicious of commercial foods and know their source.
- Grow your own food as much as you can.
- Increase consumption of fruits, vegetables, and whole grains.
- For every 1,000 cal try to have at least 14 g of fiber, because fiber helps control blood sugar levels.
- Coffee and possibly tea may decrease the risk of developing DM.
- Chromium and cinnamon have been shown in some studies to improve insulin sensitivity.
- Fish oil helps in decreasing the risk of developing DM.
- Grape-seed extracts may help to decrease the risk of developing DM.
- Drink alcohol with moderation (please see Sect. 2.4).

1.11   Glaucoma

1.11.1   Risk Assessment and Prevention of Glaucoma

1.11.1.1   Risk Assessment

Genetic Markers

- There is a significant association between glaucoma and Rhesus D (+).
- There is an association between the acid phosphatase ACPC allele and primary open-angle glaucoma. It is located on chromosome 2p23. A single-nucleotide polymorphism (SNP) on intervening sequence (IVS) 8 (IVS8+4 C/T) is strongly associated with the occurrence of normal-tension glaucoma, and it is located on the OPA1 gene.
- The myocilin/TIGR gene (GLC1A) is responsible for about 4 % of the cases of glaucoma. It can be useful when there is a suspected family history since patients with this genetic marker tend to have rapidly developing glaucoma and should be treated more aggressively. It also tends to be more commonly associated with glaucoma under the age of 40.
- The WDR36 (GLC1G) gene has mutations that appear to be associated with glaucoma.
- The optineurin gene (GLC1E) is associated with an increased incidence of glaucoma in patients with normal pressures.
- A form of juvenile open-angle glaucoma has been clearly linked to genetic abnormalities.
- One uncommon form of glaucoma known as pseudoexfoliation glaucoma has also seen the development of a genetic marker test.
- Less than 10 % of glaucomas have a direct genetic cause.
- Please see Table in *Arch Ophthalmol* (2007);125(1):30–37. doi:10.1001/archopht.125.1.30, via the following link: http://archopht.jamanetwork.com/article.aspx?articleid=418917.

Biochemical and Serological Markers

- Oxidative stress may lead to an induction of antioxidant enzymes and contribute to TRAP decrease. Superoxide dismutase, GPx activities, and TRAP may be useful oxidative stress markers in aqueous humor of glaucoma patients.

Past Medical History

- People with an elevated intraocular pressure have a higher risk of developing glaucoma, but not everyone with elevated intraocular pressure develops the disease.

- Nearsighted or farsighted people have an increased risk of developing glaucoma.
- Using corticosteroids for prolonged periods of time appears to increase the risk of developing glaucoma. This is especially true for corticosteroid eyedrops.
- Severe eye injuries can result in elevated eye pressure and increase the risk of developing glaucoma.
- Lens dislocation increases the risk of developing glaucoma.

Family History

- People with a positive family history for glaucoma are at much higher risk of developing the disease.

Comorbidities

- Retinal detachment increases the risk of developing glaucoma.
- Eye tumors increase the risk of developing glaucoma.
- Chronic uveitis and iritis increase the risk of developing glaucoma.
- Diabetes increases the risk of developing glaucoma.
- Hypothyroidism increases the risk of developing glaucoma.
- Heart diseases increase the risk of developing glaucoma.
- Suspicious optic nerve appearance (cupping >50 % or asymmetry) increases the risk of developing glaucoma.
- Central corneal thickness less than 555 μm (0.555 mm) increases the risk of developing glaucoma.
- Hypertension (maybe resulting from overweight) possibly increases the risk of developing glaucoma.
- Migraine headache and peripheral vasospasm possibly increase the risk of developing glaucoma.
- Sleep-related breathing disorder possibly increases the risk of developing glaucoma.

Age/Gender/Ethnicity/Nutrition/Lifestyle

- People older than 60 are at increased risk for developing glaucoma.
- African Americans are five times more likely to get glaucoma than Caucasians, and they are much more likely to experience permanent blindness as a result.
- Mexican Americans and Asian Americans have an increased risk of developing glaucoma.
- Men may be at higher risk of developing glaucoma than women.

Recommendations

- Eliminate/avoid/attenuate risk factors, if possible (please see above and below).
- The eyes should be periodically tested by a doctor for glaucoma as follows:
  - At 35 and 40 years of age
  - Every 4 years between 40 and 60 years of age
  - Every 1–2 years after 60 years of age
  - Every 1–2 years after 35 years of age when there are risk factors (please see above)

1.11.1.2 Preventive Advice

Chemical

- Vitamins C, E, and A protect vision.
- Zinc can be useful for protecting vision.
- Treat elevated eye pressure. Drops must be taken regularly even when there are no symptoms.

Lifestyle

- Wear eye protection, for example, when using power tools or playing high-speed racket sports on enclosed courts or whenever the eyes are at risk of being hit.
- Control blood pressure.
- Control weight. Lose weight, if necessary, by increasing caloric output through exercising (please see Sect. 2.1) and decreasing caloric input through dieting.

Nutrition

- Cod liver oil decreases intraocular pressure.

1.12 Graves' Disease

1.12.1 Risk Assessment and Prevention of Graves' Disease

1.12.1.1 Risk Assessment

Genetic Markers

- Some people may have a genetic predisposition to develop TSH receptor autoantibodies. HLADR, especially DR3, appears to play a significant role.

- There are several susceptibility genes in the regions of linkage on chromosome 2q (CTLA-4), 8q (Tg), 14q (TSHR), 20q (CD40), 5q (SCGB3A2/UGRP1), and, probably, Xp (FOXP3) linked to Graves' disease.
- Predisposing loci include 3 more genes (PTPN22, IL-2RA/CD25, and FCRL3).
- The following are some of the genes linked to Graves' disease:

Genes linked and/or associated with autoimmune thyroid disease gene symbol	Gene name	Chromosome location	Odds ratio
HLA	Major histocompatibility complex	6p21	2.0–4.0
CTLA4	Cytotoxic T-lymphocyte-associated protein 4	2q33	1.5–2.2
PTPN22	Protein tyrosine phosphatase, non-receptor type 22 (lymphoid)	1p13	1.4–1.9
CD40	CD40 molecule, TNF receptor superfamily member 5	20q11	1.3–1.8
IL-2RA (CD25)	Interleukin 2 receptor, alpha	10p15	1.1–1.4
FCRL3	Fc receptor-like 3	1q23	1.1–1.3
TG	Thyroglobulin	8q24	1.3–1.6
TSHR	Thyroid-stimulating hormone receptor	14q31	1.4–2.6

From: *J Thyroid Res* (2012) 2012, Article ID 623852, 6 pages. doi:10.1155/2012/623852

Biochemical and Serological Markers

- Thyroid peroxidase antibody (TPOAb), thyroglobulin antibody (TgAb), and thyroid-stimulating hormone receptor antibody (TRAb) are markers of Graves' disease.
- Other antibodies can be found in Graves' disease such as:

  - Elevated levels of TBII and (rarely) TSBAb
  - Antibodies reacting to the iodide symporter and pendrin protein
  - Antibodies recognizing components of the eye muscle and/or fibroblasts
  - Antibodies to DNA
  - Antibodies to parietal cells (infrequent)
  - Antibodies binding to platelets
  - Antibody Ku

- The blood tests for Graves' disease are in Table 1.28.

Past Medical History

- Pregnancy or recent childbirth (especially the first year after delivery) increases the risk of developing Graves' disease (particularly in women who are genetically susceptible).
- Some treatments and medications can trigger Graves' disease, including interferon beta-1b and interleukin-4, immunosuppressant therapy, antiretroviral treatment for AIDS, and lithium.

Table 1.28   Testing for Graves' disease

TSH blood test	Lower than normal levels of TSH indicate hyperthyroidism or Graves' disease
T4 and T3 blood tests	High levels of thyroxine and triiodothyronine may indicate hyperthyroidism
Graves' antibody test	The presence of antibodies in the blood is associated with Graves' disease

- Two particular treatments are known triggers for Graves' disease: (1) a third of patients receiving monoclonal antibody (Campath-1H) therapy for multiple sclerosis (MS) develop Graves' disease within 6 months and (2) receiving a donated organ or bone marrow transplant from someone with Graves' disease can cause the disease in the recipient.
- Use of sex steroids increases the risk of developing Graves' disease.
- Radiation to the neck can trigger Graves' disease.

Family History

- Family history of Graves' disease (or autoimmune disorder) is a risk factor for developing the disease.
- The concordance rate for Graves' disease among homozygotic twins is 35 % but much lower in dizygotic twins.

Comorbidities

- Graves' disease is associated with pernicious anemia, vitiligo, diabetes mellitus type 1, autoimmune adrenal insufficiency, systemic sclerosis, myasthenia gravis, Sjögren syndrome, rheumatoid arthritis, and systemic lupus erythematosus.
- Viral infections can trigger Graves' disease.

Age/Gender/Ethnicity/Nutrition/Lifestyle

- Graves' disease affects women five to ten times more often than men.
- The riskiest age for developing Graves' disease is between 20 and 40 years old.
- Emotionally or physically stressful life events or illnesses may be triggers for Graves' disease for people who are genetically susceptible.
- Cigarette smoking increases the risk of developing Graves' disease. Risk increase is proportional to the number of cigarettes smoked daily.
- Even a minimal amount of weekly alcohol consumption (one bottle of beer or one glass of wine per week) appears to reduce the risk of Graves' diseases independent of age, sex, smoking, and comorbidities. This effect is greater with moderate consumption.
- Copper deficiency may be associated with Graves' disease.
- Obesity decreases the risk of developing Graves' disease.

Recommendations

- Eliminate/avoid/attenuate risk factors, if possible (please see above and below).
- The American Thyroid Association recommends TSH screening every 5 years for individuals above age 35.
- In women, thyroid gland function should be assessed as part of routine physical checkups.

1.12.1.2   Preventive Advice

Chemical

- Selenium may prevent the progression of autoimmune thyroid disease.
- L-Carnitine has an impact on hyperfunctioning thyroid glands.
- If there is a copper deficiency, supplements should be taken to prevent Graves' disease.

Lifestyle

- Exercise (please see Sect. 2.1).
- Ease stress as much as possible (please see Sect. 2.2).
- Do not smoke/quit smoking or chewing tobacco (please see Sect. 2.3).

Nutrition

- Eat a balanced diet. The Stanford Health Improvement Program recommends the Mediterranean diet.
- Drink alcohol with moderation (please see Sect. 2.4).

1.13   Hemochromatosis (Primary/HFE Related)

1.13.1   Risk Assessment and Prevention of Primary Hemochromatosis (HFE Related)

1.13.1.1   Risk Assessment

Genetic Markers

- Hemochromatosis is linked to the HFE gene. The protein product of the HFE gene is a transmembrane glycoprotein called HFE that modulates iron uptake. Mutations in the HFE protein compromise its function and produce disease symptoms. Two mutations, C282Y and H63D, have been linked to the majority of hemochromatosis cases.

- Having two copies of a mutated HFE gene is the greatest risk factor for hereditary hemochromatosis.
- However, many people who have two copies of the faulty gene do not develop signs or symptoms of the disease.
- There are two well-known alleles of the hemochromatosis (HFE) gene, designated C282Y and H63D, in addition to the normal version of the gene. The disease symptoms and the age of onset depend on which combination of alleles a person has inherited.
- Please see Table 1.29 for the hemochromatosis genes and proteins.

Biochemical and Serological Markers

- Please see Table 1.30.

Table 1.29   The hemochromatosis genes and proteins

Gene	Protein	Protein class	Expression	Interaction	Disease type by OMIM
HFE	HFE	HLA class I, atypical	Ubiquitous	TFR1	1
TFR2	TFR2	TFR family	Hepatocytes	Transferrin	3
HAMP	Hepcidin	Antimicrobial peptide	Hepatocytes, skeletal muscle, heart	Ferroportin	2b
HJV	Hemojuvelin	RGM homologue	Heart, liver, skeletal muscle	Neogenin	2a
SLC40A1	Ferroportin	Iron exporter	Ubiquitous	Hepcidin	4

From: *Blood* (2005) 106(12):3710–3371
OMIM Online Mendelian Inheritance in Man101, *HJV* hemojuvelin-encoding gene, *SLC40A1* solute carrier family 40, member 1, *HLA* human leukocyte antigen, *TFR1* transferrin receptor 1, *RGM* repulsive guidance molecule

Table 1.30   Hemochromatosis blood values

Serum	Normal	Hereditary hemochromatosis
Iron		
(mug/dL)	60–180	180–300
(mumol/L)	11–32	32–54
Transferrin saturation (%)[a]	20–50	55–100
Ferritin		
Males (ng/mL; mug/L)	20–200	300–3,000
Females (ng/mL; mug/L)	15–150	250–3,000

From: http://articles.mercola.com/sites/articles/archive/2002/12/18/iron-diagnosis.aspx#_edn7
[a]Unsaturated-iron binding capacity is an inexpensive alternative to percent transferring saturation. The optimum threshold for detection is 143 microg/dL (25.6 micromol/L, giving a sensitivity of 0.91 and a specificity of 0.95)

Family History

- People with a close relative (grandparent, mother, father, sibling, niece, nephew) presenting hemochromatosis have a higher chance of having the HFE gene mutation.

Comorbidities

- People with hemochromatosis are susceptible to infections, especially those caused by certain bacteria in raw shellfish.
- People with hemochromatosis have an increased risk of developing heart failure.
- People with hemochromatosis have an increased risk of developing diabetes.
- People with hemochromatosis have an increased risk of developing cirrhosis.
- People with hemochromatosis have an increased risk of developing liver cancer.

Age/Gender/Ethnicity/Nutrition/Lifestyle

- Men are at higher risk for developing hemochromatosis than women.
- Older people are more likely to develop the disease than younger ones. Signs and symptoms usually do not occur in men until 40–60 years of age.
- In women, signs and symptoms usually do not occur before menopause.
- Young children rarely develop hemochromatosis.
- People of Northern European descent are at higher risk for developing hemochromatosis.
- Hemochromatosis is less common in African Americans, Hispanics, and Asian Americans.
- Alcoholism is a risk factor for developing hemochromatosis.

Recommendations

- Eliminate/avoid/attenuate risk factors, if possible (please see above and below).
- The following are the CDC recommended guidelines for hemochromatosis:

Genetic Markers

- *All first-degree relatives of subjects known to have hemochromatosis*: Human leukocyte antigen (HLA) typing is no longer necessary; family members identified as having C282Y homozygosity should be tested for transferrin saturation, serum ferritin, and liver enzymes; screening of young children of patients with hemochromatosis does not need to be performed if the spouse is tested and does not have the C282Y mutation.

- *Individuals presenting for a standard medical check*: Transferrin saturation should be measured; if levels are higher than 45 %, the estimation should be repeated after fasting—if the fasting level still is higher than 45 %, further investigation is warranted.
- *The general population*: This group possibly should be screened, although screening is more difficult and debatable in these individuals and cost is a major consideration; a consensus stated that population screening is best performed by phenotype (using iron-binding capacity), but genotype screening (using C282Y mutation) is premature until all unanswered questions are clarified.
- *If a proband is negative for C282Y mutation*: Family members must be screened by other means, such as serum iron studies or HLA typing; HLA typing or tissue typing has been used to detect homozygous hemochromatosis in a sibling of a proband who has hemochromatosis by liver biopsy or quantitative phlebotomy—in this setting, a sibling who is HLA-A and HLA-B identical to the proband is considered homozygous; if only 1 haplotype is shared with the proband, the sibling is considered heterozygous.

Beyond Genetic Markers

Other tests include:

- Blood measurements of serum transferrin saturation and serum ferritin
- A liver biopsy, if necessary
- An MRI, if necessary

1.13.1.2   Preventive Advice

Chemical

- Avoid iron supplements and multivitamins containing iron, if at risk for hemochromatosis.
- Avoid vitamin C supplements (vitamin C increases absorption of iron), if at risk for hemochromatosis.

Nutrition

The following diet is recommended for people at risk for hemochromatosis:

- Avoid red meat (rich in iron).
- Avoid sugars that can increase iron absorption and free radical cell damage.
- Increase intake of substances that inhibit iron absorption, such as high-tannin tea and calcium.
- Eat foods containing oxalic and phytic acids such as collard greens, which must be consumed at the same time as the iron-containing foods in order to be effective.

- Eat fresh fruits and vegetables that provide antioxidants, vitamins, minerals, and fiber.
- Snack on fruit or carrots, when energy is needed.
- Add extra vegetables (kale, bok choy, carrot) to salads.
- Use whole-grain cereal at breakfast.
- Eat nuts.
- Eat whole, unprocessed food.
- Limit diary foods.
- Limit animal fat.
- Limit intake of alcoholic beverages (please see Sect. 2.4).

1.14   Lactose Intolerance

1.14.1   Risk Assessment and Prevention of Lactose Intolerance

1.14.1.1   Risk Assessment

Genetic Markers

- Lactase production is controlled by an autosomal gene, located on chromosome 2.
- Persistence of lactase production is a dominant trait in lactose intolerance.
- There are 2 alleles, designated LAC*P for lactase persistence and LAC*R for normal adult lactase restriction. The LAC locus appears to be a regulatory gene that decreases lactase synthesis by reducing the transcription of messenger RNA. Persons inheriting LAC*P from both parents have lactase persistence into adulthood; those getting LAC*R alleles from both parents display lactase restriction as adults.
- Heterozygotes get different alleles and are LAC*P/LAC*R, but since LAC*P is dominant, lactase activity and ability to digest milk persist beyond childhood.
- Investigators have identified a genetic variant or SNP (C/T13910), 14 kb upstream of the LCH (lactase–phlorizin hydrolase) locus on the large arm of human chromosome 2 (2q21).

Biochemical and Serological Markers

- The stool acidity test is usually performed on infants or small children who are not eligible for other tests. A stool sample is taken to see if lactose has been broken properly in the GI tract. Fermenting lactose (a sign of lactose intolerance) creates lactic acid, which can be detected in stool.
- For adult tests, please see Table 1.31.

Table 1.31 Summary of tests for lactose malabsorption and tolerance

	H$_2$-breath test	Lactose tolerance test	Genetic test of −13910 C/T polymorphism	Lactase activity at jejunal brush border
Test principle	Increase of H$_2$ in respiratory air after lactose challenge	Increase of blood sugar after lactose challenge	Genetic Polymorphism 13910 upstream of lactase gene	Enzymatic activity of lactase enzyme in biopsy sample
Cut off	>20 ppm within 3 h	<1.1 mmol/L within 3 h	13910C/C indicates lactase non-persistence	<17–20 IU/g
Availability	Good	Excellent	Variable	Rare
False positives (malabsorption incorrectly diagnosed)	Rapid GI-transit, small-intestinal bacterial overgrowth	Rapid GI-transit, impaired glucose tolerance	Rare (<5 %) in Caucasians	Probably rare
False negatives (malabsorption wrongly excluded)	Non-H$_2$-producers. Full colonic adaptation.	Fluctuations in blood sugar	All causes of secondary lactose malabsorption	Patchy enzyme expression
Secondary causes	Cannot be excluded, kinetic of H$_2$-increase can be suggestive	Cannot be excluded	Cannot be excluded	Can be excluded (histopathology obtained at same procedure)
Assessment of symptoms/ lactose tolerance	Possible	Possible	Not possible	Not possible
Comment	Method of choice for assessment of lactose malabsorption and intolerance	Rarely performed due to inferior sensitivity and specificity	Definitive test for lactase non-persistence in Caucasians. Less suitable in other populations. Not suitable in patients with intestinal disease at risk of secondary lactase deficiency.	Reference standard for detection of lactase deficiency (primary or secondary)
Cost	Low	Lowest	High	Highest

From: *United European Gastroenterology J* (2013)

Past Medical History

- Prematurity increases the risk of developing lactose intolerance.
- Radiation therapy for cancer in the abdomen increases the risk of developing lactose intolerance.

Family History

- A family history of lactose intolerance increases the risk of developing the disease.

Comorbidities

- Diseases affecting the small intestine such as bacterial overgrowth, celiac disease, and Crohn's disease increase the risk of developing lactose intolerance.

Age/Gender/Ethnicity/Nutrition/Lifestyle

- The risk of developing lactose intolerance increases with age.
- Lactose intolerance is uncommon in babies and young children.
- 95 % of Asians, 60–80 % of African Americans and Ashkenazi Jews, 80–100 % of American Indians, and 50–80 % of Hispanics have lactose intolerance. It is least common in people of North European origin (2–5 %). Please see Table 1.32.

Recommendations

- Eliminate/avoid/attenuate risk factors (please see above and below).
- If there is a suspicion of lactose intolerance, screening tests must be prescribed (please see above).

1.14.1.2 Preventive Advice

Nutrition

- There are no means of preventing lactose intolerance, in particular avoiding milk completely for long periods of time does not lead to a change in lactase production.

Table 1.32 Lactose
intolerance

Population	Hypolactasia prevalence (%)
Southeast Asians	98
Asian Americans	90
Alaskan Eskimo	80
African American adults	79
Mexicans (rural communities)	74
North American Jews	69
Greek Cypriots	66
Cretans	56
Mexican American males	55
Indian Adults	50
African American children	45
Indian children	20
Descendants of N. Europeans	5

From: http://nutrigenomics.ucdavis.edu/?page=information/
Concepts_in_Nutrigenomics/Lactose_Intolerance

1.15   Lung Cancer

1.15.1   Risk Assessment and Prevention of Lung Cancer

1.15.1.1   Risk Assessment

Genetic Markers

- The LCS6 variant allele in a *KRAS* miRANA complementary site is significantly associated with increased risk for NSCLC (non-small cell lung cancer) among moderate smokers and represents a new paradigm for *let-7* miRNAs in lung cancer susceptibility.
- The GSTM1 null genotype is greatest in female smokers, which is consistent with other evidence that indicates that women are at higher risk of lung cancer than males, given equal smoking.
- Persons with both the GSTM1 deletion and elevated PAH-DNA adducts may represent a sensitive subpopulation with respect to carcinogens in tobacco smoke and other environmental media.
- P450CYPIA genotype type C is strongly associated with lung cancer.
- Specific genotype combinations of the CYPIA1, GSTM1, and GSTT1 alleles are involved in the development of lung cancer in heavy smokers.
- Several SNPs are associated with lung cancer (Please see Table 1.33).

Biochemical and Serological Markers

- Please see Table 1.34 for comparison of diagnostic results of NAB alone and NAB combined with tumor markers according to histological subtype.

Table 1.33 Association between SNPs and lung cancer

SNP	PHWE	Frequency of high-risk allele	Observed OR, (95 % CI)[a]	p	Genetic variance explained[b]
rs2736100	0.49	0.41	1.18 (1.09–1.27)	<0.001	1.33 %
rs402710	0.43	0.68	1.10 (1.01–1.19)	0.034	0.40 %
rs1051730	0.05	0.02	1.09 (0.85–1.40)	0.108	–
rs4083914	0.25	0.14	1.15 (1.03–1.28)	0.013	0.47 %
rs4488809	0.50	0.47	1.21 (1.11–1.30)	<0.001	1.82 %

From: *BMC Med Genet* (2012) 13:118. doi:10.1186/1471-2350-13-118
Note: *CI* confidence interval, *OR* odds ratio
[a]Odds ratio per copy of the high-risk allele
[b]The percentage of genetic variance was estimated under a liability threshold model: $[2p (1-p)] \beta2$ (p, risk allele frequency; β, additive allelic effect)

Table 1.34 Comparison of diagnostic results of NAB alone and NAB combined with tumor markers according to histological subtype

Diagnostic method	Sensitivity (%)	Specificity (%)	Accuracy (%)	PPV (%)	NPV (%)
Adenocarcinoma subtype (n=92)					
NAB alone	79.3	100	87.1	100	74.3
NAB+serum tumor marker					
CYFRA (3.3)	81.5	81.8	81.6	88.2	72.6
CEA (5)	81.5	90.9	85	93.8	74.6
SCC (2)	79.3	92.7	84.4	94.8	72.9
NAB+cytological tumor marker					
CYFRA (15.7)	92.4	98.2	94.6	98.8	88.5
CEA (0.6)	89.1	92.7	90.5	95.3	83.6
SCC (0.86)	83.5	70.9	81.6	88	78
Squamous cell carcinoma subtype (n=29)					
NAB alone	89.7	100	96.4	100	94.8
NAB+serum tumor marker					
CYFRA (3.3)	93.1	81.8	85.7	73	95.7
CEA (5)	93.1	90.9	91.7	84.4	96.2
SCC (2)	93.1	92.7	92.9	87.1	96.2
NAB+cytological tumor marker					
CYFRA (15.7)	100	98.2	98.8	96.7	100
CEA (0.6)	96.6	92.7	94	87.5	98.1
SCC (0.86)	100	70.9	81	64.4	100

From: *BMC Cancer* (2012) 12:392. doi:10.1186/1471-2407-12-392
Note: Numbers in parentheses are cutoff levels of tumor markers in ng/mL
Abbreviations: *PPV* positive predictive value, *NPV* negative predictive value, *CEA* carcinoembryonic antigen, *SCC* squamous cell carcinoma, *CYFRA* cytokeratin 19 fragments, *NAB* needle aspiration biopsy

Past Medical History

- Survivors of lung cancer have a greater risk than the general population of developing a second lung cancer. Their risk for development of second cancers approaches 6 % per year. However, survivors of non-small cell lung cancers have an additive risk of 1–2 % per year for developing a second lung cancer.
- Cancer treatments, like radiation therapy, increase the risk of developing lung cancer.
- A history of lung disease may increase the risk of developing lung cancer.
- Recent evidence suggests that some viruses may increase the risk of developing lung cancer such as HPV and CMV.

Family History

- People with a parent, sibling, or child with lung cancer have an increased risk of developing the disease.

Comorbidities

- Smokers with certain lung diseases, such as emphysema, may have an increased risk of developing lung cancer.

Age/Gender/Ethnicity/Nutrition/Lifestyle

- With the same amount of cigarettes smoked, women are at higher risk than men for developing lung cancer.
- In the United States, cigarette smoking causes about 90 % of lung cancers.
- The risk of lung cancer increases with the number of cigarettes smoked daily and the number of years of smoking.
- People who quit smoking have a lower risk of lung cancer than if they had continued to smoke, but their risk is higher than the risk for people who never smoked.
- Exposure to secondhand smoke increases the risk of developing lung cancer.
- Exposure to radon gas increases the risk of developing lung cancer.
- Exposure to asbestos and other chemicals such as arsenic, chromium, nickel or to soot or tar increases the risk of developing lung cancer, especially in smokers.
- Air pollution including diesel exhaust increases the risk of developing lung cancer.
- Drinking more than a moderate amount of alcohol may increase the risk of developing lung cancer.

- Excess body weight seems to be inversely associated with squamous cell carcinoma and adenocarcinoma.
- Total and recreational physical activity reduces lung cancer risk by 20–30 % for women and 20–50 % for men, and there is evidence of a dose–response effect.

Recommendations

- Eliminate/avoid/attenuate risk factors, if possible (please see above and below).
- Do not smoke/quit smoking, at any age.
- Calculate lung cancer risk: http://www.hellohaveyouheard.com/lung-cancer-risk-assessment/.

1.15.1.2 Preventive Advice

Chemical

- Beta-carotene may help prevent lung cancer.
- Avoid taking large doses of vitamin supplements.

Lifestyle

- Know about lung cancer (please see Sect. 2.12).
- Do not smoke/quit smoking (please see Sect. 2.3).
- Avoid secondhand smoke.
- Avoid carcinogens, if applicable.
- Get regular exercise (please see Sect. 2.1).

Nutrition

- Foods high in lutein such as collard greens, spinach, broccoli, and orange juice are associated with a lower risk of lung cancer.
- Foods high in lycopene such as tomatoes and especially tomato sauces are linked to a lower risk of lung cancer.
- Eating at least two servings of fruits each day leads to reduced risk of developing lung cancer (particularly apples).
- Drink alcohol with moderation (please see Sect. 2.4).
- Smokers who drink green tea appear to have decreased oxidative DNA damage, a genetic change that predisposes to cancer.

1.16   Lupus Erythematosus (Systemic)

1.16.1   Risk Assessment and Prevention of Systemic Lupus Erythematosus (SLE)

1.16.1.1   Risk Assessment

Genetic Markers

- Two genes from the interferon system, IRF5 and STAT4, and the HLA system are the three strongest risk factors for SLE.
- The most important genes are located in the HLA region on chromosome 6, where mutations may occur randomly or may be inherited.
- HLA class I, class II, and class III are associated with SLE, but only classes I and II contribute independently to increased risk.
- Other genes which contain risk variants for SLE are PTPN22, STAT4, CDK1A, TNFSF4, and BANK1. Some of the susceptibility genes may be population specific, for example, in African Americans, SLEH1 at 11q14 is associated with an increased risk of developing SLE.
- BLK and ITGAM are genes associated with an increased risk of developing SLE.
- There are 40 genetic biomarkers of lupus which are microRNAs in cell nuclei.
- For example, the 3′-untranslated region (3′-UTR) of the CTLA4 gene is involved in susceptibility to SLE.
- Please see table in *Nature Reviews Genetics*, 10, 285-290 (May 2009), via the following link:
- http://www.nature.com/nrg/journal/v10/n5/full/nrg2571.html.

Biochemical and Serological Markers

- *Hematologic disorder*: hemolytic anemia with reticulocytosis, or leukopenia <4,000 per mm^3 (4.0×10^9 per L) on two or more occasions, or lymphopenia <1,500 per mm^3 (1.5×10^9 per L) on two or more occasions, or thrombocytopenia <100 × 10^3 per mm^3 (100×10^9 per L) in the absence of offending drugs.
- *Immunologic disorder*: antibody to double-stranded DNA antigen (anti-dsDNA) in abnormal titer; or presence of antibody to Sm nuclear antigen (anti-Sm); or positive finding of antiphospholipid antibody based on an abnormal serum level of IgG or IgM anticardiolipin antibodies, a positive test result for lupus anticoagulant using a standard method, or a false-positive serologic test for syphilis that is known to be positive for at least 6 months and is confirmed by negative *Treponema pallidum* immobilization or fluorescent treponemal antibody absorption test.

Table 1.35 30 protein analytes dysregulated in SLE serum

Analyte	All SLE v Ctrl FC		SLE IFN-hi v Ctrl FC		SLE IFN-lo v Ctrl FC		SLE IFN-hi v IFN-lo FC	
IFN-ω	-1.88	***	-1.87	***	-1.89	***	1.01	
ACE	-1.34	**	-1.55	***	-1.18		-1.32	
FGF RIII	-1.48	**	-1.50	*	-1.46	*	-1.02	
ACE-2	-1.09		-1.46	**	1.15		-1.68	*
PDGF-RA	-1.50	***	-1.46	**	-1.55	***	1.06	
CCL20 (MIP-3A)	-1.48	**	-1.43	*	-1.53	**	1.06	
FGF-2	-1.41	***	-1.34	*	-1.50	***	1.12	
GDNF	1.43	***	1.53	**	1.33	*	1.15	
BDNF	1.21		1.55	*	-1.14		1.76	*
ICAM3	1.31	**	1.56	**	1.07		1.46	*
CXCL11 (I-TAC)	1.23		1.58	*	-1.15		1.81	*
CCL7 (MCP-3)	1.57	*****	1.63	***	1.51	**	1.08	
MMP7	1.58	**	1.64	**	1.53		1.07	
IL-18	1.46	**	1.71	**	1.22		1.40	*
IL-5	1.54	***	1.72	**	1.37	*	1.26	
CCL17 (TARC)	1.61	*	1.74	*	1.48		1.17	
IL-2SRA	1.71	****	1.81	**	1.61	**	1.12	
IL-15	1.58	**	1.88	*	1.28	***	1.47	
CCL3 (MIP-1A)	1.69	*****	2.00	*****	1.38	**	1.45	***
CXCL2 (GROB)	1.82	*	2.13	*	1.52		1.40	
EGF	2.12	**	2.16	**	2.08	*	1.04	
CXCL13 (BLC)	1.96	***	2.18	**	1.73		1.26	
TGF-B RIII	2.18	**	2.34	**	2.02	*	1.15	
CXCL8 (IL-8)	2.31	****	2.49	**	2.14	**	1.16	
CCL19 (MIP-3B)	2.05	***	2.82	****	1.27		2.22	***
IL-6	2.83	*****	3.11	****	2.55	**	1.22	
CXCL9 (MIG)	2.29	*	3.24	*	1.34		2.42	*
CCL8 (MCP-2)	2.48	****	3.27	***	1.69	*	1.93	*
CCL2 (MCP-1)	3.78	***	5.52	**	2.04		2.71	*
CXCL10 (IP-10)	5.82	**	9.09	**	1.74	*	5.82	**

From: http://www.plosmedicine.org/article/info%3Adoi%2F10.1371%2Fjournal.pmed.0030491

- *Antinuclear antibodies*: an abnormal antinuclear antibody titer by immunofluorescence or equivalent assay at any time and in the absence of drugs known to be associated with drug-induced lupus.
- Thirty protein analytes dysregulated in SLE serum are in Table 1.35.

Past Medical History

- More than 38 medications can cause SLE. The most common are procainamide, isoniazid, quinidine, and phenytoin.

Family History

- An identical twin of a person with lupus has a threefold to tenfold greater risk of developing SLE than a nonidentical twin.
- First-degree relatives of people with lupus have an eightfold to ninefold increased risk of developing SLE compared with the general population.

Similarly:

- Autoimmune diseases such as rheumatoid arthritis and autoimmune thyroid disorders are more common among relatives of people with SLE than the general population.

Comorbidities

- SLE may occur with other autoimmune conditions (e.g., thyroiditis, hemolytic anemia, idiopathic thrombocytopenic purpura).
- Some infectious agents may increase the risk of developing SLE (viruses, bacteria, fungi).

Similarly:

- People with SLE are at increased risk for developing cancers such as leukemia and lymphoma.

Age/Gender/Ethnicity/Nutrition/Lifestyle

- SLE is six to ten times more common in women.
- SLE is most often diagnosed between the ages of 15 and 40.
- SLE is more common in African Americans, Hispanics, and Asians.
- Certain toxins and diets have been linked to the development of SLE.
- Sun exposure (ultraviolet light) can worsen rashes of patients with SLE and sometimes trigger a flare of the entire disease.

Recommendations

- Eliminate/avoid/attenuate risk factors, if possible (please see above and below).
- Ruling out SLE is sometimes difficult. Physicians use 11 different criteria to make its diagnosis.

1.16.1.2 Preventive Advice

Chemical

- Vitamin D may help prevent SLE.

Lifestyle

- Exercise regularly (please see Sect. 2.1).
- Get adequate rest (please see Sect. 2.2).
- Decrease stress (please see Sect. 2.2). Several studies have shown that meditation can reduce stress-induced immune responses.
- Do not smoke/quit smoking or chewing tobacco (please see Sect. 2.3).

Nutrition

- Eat a healthy diet emphasizing fruits, vegetables, and whole grains.
- The following nutrients may help prevent SLE:

  - Flaxseed
  - Fish oil

1.17   Macular Degeneration (Age Related)

1.17.1   Risk Assessment and Prevention of Age-Related Macular Degeneration (AMD)

1.17.1.1   Risk Assessment

Genetic Markers

- Single-nucleotide polymorphisms in complement factor H (CFH) and PLEKHA1/ARMS2/HtrA1 capture a substantial fraction of AMD risk and permit the identification of individuals at high risk for developing AMD. Please see Table 1.36.
- A powerful predictor of AMD is on chromosome 10q26 at LOC 387715.

Similarly:

- Other gene markers of disease progression risk include tissue inhibitor of metalloproteinase 3.
- Variations in cholesterol metabolizing genes such as hepatic lipase, cholesterol ester transferase, lipoprotein lipase, and the ABC-binding cassette A1 correlate with disease progression.

Biochemical and Serological Markers

- High cholesterol is associated with an increased risk of developing AMD.
- Elevated plasma fibrinogen moderately increases the risk of developing AMD.
- Please see Table 1.37 for complement proteins in AMD.

Table 1.36 Summary of conclusions from meta-analysis of established associations (three or more published reports) between AMD and genetic variants

Gene	Polymorphism	Total studies	Total (N)	Allele	Cases	Controls	Odds ratio	Meta-analysis (p value)
					Allele frequencies			
CFH	**rs1061170** (C/T)	14	10 930	T	0.435	0.639	2.00	$<10^{-100}$
LOC387715	**rs10490924** (G/T)	8	8,473	T	0.420	0.207	2.62	$<10^{-100}$
C2	**rs9332739** (C/G)	4	4,184	G	0.977	0.943	2.42	1.0×10^{-12}
C2	**rs547154 (A/C)**	4	4,162	C	0.949	0.892	2.20	6.8×10^{-10}
BF	**rs4151667** (A/T)	4	4,197	T	0.974	0.942	2.20	9.5×10^{-11}
ApoE	–	8	4,290	ε2	0.097	0.076	1.33	0.042
				ε3	0.808	0.784	1.28	0.00024
				ε4	0.095	0.152	0.60	1.7×10^{-11}

From: *Hum Mol Genet* (2007) 16(R2):R174–R182. doi:10.1093/hmg/ddm212

Table 1.37 Median plasma concentrations of complement proteins in age-related macular degeneration and control subjects and the impact on risk for having AMD

Protein	AMD Median	AMD Percentiles (25th, 75th)	Control Median	Control Percentiles (25th, 75th)	Uncorrected p value[a]	Corrected and standardized Odds ratio[b] (95 % confidence interval)	p value[b]
Factor B (μg/ml)	1,103	(931, 1,381)	985	(823, 1174)	0.01	1.22 (0.94–1.60)	0.13
Factor D (μg/ml)	1.50	(1.20, 1.91)	1.16	(0.96, 1.47)	0.00003	1.57 (1.17–2.15)	0.004
FH/FHR-1 (μg/ml)[c]	681	(625, 769)	668	(591, 757)	0.44	1.17 (0.92–1.50)	0.19
C5a (ng/ml)	4.28	(3.04, 5.40)	4.06	(2.39, 5.19)	0.36	1.14 (0.89–1.46)	0.30
Ba (μg/ml)	1.07	(0.80, 1.67)	0.78	(0.62, 1.02)	0.0001	1.69 (1.27–2.33)	0.0006
C3d (μg/ml)	40.7	(31.8, 47.7)	35.8	(30.2, 43.0)	0.002	1.43 (1.11–1.89)	0.009

From: *Hum Mol Genet* (2010) 19(1):209–215

[a]*P* value for difference in "raw" median plasma levels without correction

[b]Odds ratios and *p* values for the effect of an increase of 1 SD in the corrected and standardized plasma level for each protein. For example, an increase of 1 SD of Ba increased the odds of having AMD by 1.69-fold

[c]Combined levels of factor H (FH) and factor H related-1 (FHR-1) were determined

Past Medical History

- Previous cataract surgery strongly increases the risk of developing AMD.
- Diseases that affect the cardiovascular system, such as high blood pressure, moderately increase the risk of developing AMD.
- Some cases of macular degeneration can be induced by drugs such as chloroquine or phenothiazine.

Family History

- A positive family history for AMD strongly increases the risk of developing the disease.

Comorbidities

- Renal disease can increase the risk of developing AMD.
- Alzheimer's disease can increase the risk of developing AMD.
- Myocardial infarction can increase the risk of developing AMD.
- Stroke can increase the risk of developing AMD.
- Diabetes mellitus can increase the risk of developing AMD.
- Arthritis can increase the risk of developing AMD.

    Similarly:

- AMD is associated with cancer (e.g., in African Americans, early AMD is associated with a fivefold higher risk of lung cancer death).

Age/Gender/Ethnicity/Nutrition/Lifestyle

- The risk of developing AMD increases with age. Macular degeneration is most common in people over 60.
- AMD is more common in Caucasians.
- Women are more likely than men to develop AMD.
- Smoking cigarettes strongly increases the risk of developing AMD.
- People living with a smoker double their risk of developing AMD.
- The risks for early age-related macular degeneration (AMD) and wet late AMD are associated with frequent aspirin use, and the risk increases with greater aspirin consumption.
- Overweight patients with macular degeneration have more than double the risk of developing advanced forms of the disease.
- A diet that includes few fruits and vegetables may increase the risk of developing AMD.

Recommendations

- Eliminate/avoid/attenuate risk factors, if possible (please see above and below).
- Check vision regularly with the Amsler grid.
- Viewing the Amsler grid separately with each eye helps monitor vision loss. The Amsler grid is a very sensitive test and, it may reveal central vision problems before AMD-related damage to the macula can be seen in a routine eye exam.

1.17.1.2 Preventive Advice

Chemical

- Avoid frequent aspirin use.
- If at risk for AMD, avoid some drugs such as chloroquine and phenothiazine.
- Many researchers and eye care practitioners believe that some antioxidants and mineral nutrients such as zinc, lutein, zeaxanthin and vitamins A, C, and E and others help lower the risk of AMD. For example, some recommend a daily intake of:
  - 500 mg of vitamin C
  - 400 international units of vitamin E
  - 15 mg of beta-carotene (equivalent of 25,000 international units of vitamin A)
  - 80 mg of zinc as zinc oxide
  - 2 mg of copper as cupric oxide

Lifestyle

- Get regular exercise (please see Sect. 2.1).
- Do not smoke/quit smoking or chewing tobacco (please see Sect. 2.3).
- Avoid secondhand smoke.
- Be lean (calculate BMI and lose weight, if necessary, by increasing caloric output through exercising and decreasing caloric intake through dieting).
- Manage diseases. For example, keep blood pressure and blood sugar under control.

Nutrition

- Choose a healthy diet full of a variety of fruits and vegetables.
- Control cholesterol (please see Sect. 2.7). The Stanford Health Improvement Program recommends the Mediterranean diet. Omega-3 fatty acids, which

Table 1.38 Foods with lutein and zeaxanthin

Food	Serving	mg
Kale (*cooked*)	1 cup	23.8
Spinach (*cooked*)	1 cup	20.4
Collards (*cooked*)	1 cup	14.6
Turnip greens (*cooked*)	1 cup	12.2
Spinach (*raw*)	1 cup	3.8
Corn (*can or cooked*)	1 cup	2.2
Green peas (*canned*)	1 cup	2.2
Broccoli (*cooked*)	1 cup	1.6
Romaine lettuce (*raw*)	1 cup	1.3
Green beans (*cooked*)	1 cup	0.8
Eggs	2 (*large*)	0.3
Orange	1 (*medium*)	0.2

are found in fish and nuts may reduce the risk of dry macular degeneration.

- Healthy unsaturated fats, such as those found in olive oil, may help protect vision.
- Avoid saturated fats found in butter and trans fats such as partially hydrogenated oils found in packaged foods.
- Prefer whole grains such as whole-wheat bread to refined grains such as white bread.
- Eat foods containing lutein and zeaxanthin. Please see Table 1.38.

1.18 Melanoma

1.18.1 Risk Assessment and Prevention of Melanoma

1.18.1.1 Risk Assessment

Genetic Markers

- More than 100 studies have proposed gene alterations that may be associated with the risk of developing melanoma.
- At least eight loci have been identified as being associated with a risk of developing melanoma ($p < .05$), of which four loci showed a genome-wide statistically significant association ($p < 1 \times 10(-7)$, including 16q24.3 (MC1R), 20q11.22 (MYH7B/PIGU/ASIP), 11q14.3 (TYR), and 5p13.2 (SLC45A2) as well as one additional gene at 9p23 (TYRP1).
- A locus at 9p21.3, CDKN2A/MTAP increases the risk of developing melanoma. Please see Table 1.39, for melanoma-associated genetic variants.

Table 1.39 Melanoma-associated genetic variants

Location	Potential gene	Genome-wide significant	MelGene score	MelGene OR	Top SNPs	GWAS OR	Pigmentation	Nevus	Independent association with melanoma
1q42	PARP1	Yes	NA	NA	rs3219090	0.89	Weak	Weak	Yes
1q21	Multitude	Yes	NA	NA	rs7412746	0.90	No	No	Yes
2q33.1	CASP8	Yes	NA	NA	rs13016963	1.14 (1.09, 1.19)	No	Weak	Yes
5p13.3–13.2	SLC45A2	Yes	A	0.4 (0.33, 0.47)	rs16891982	0.36 (0.23, 0.53)	Yes	No	No
5p15.33	TERT	Yes	B	0.87 (1.15, 1.22)	rs401681	0.87 (0.81, 0.94)	No	Weak	Yes
9p21.3	CDKN2A	Yes	C, HWE violated	1.25 (1.03, 1.51)	Multiple	0.83 (0.78, 0.88)	No	Weak	Yes
9p21.3	MTAP	Yes	A	~0.81 to ~0.84	Multiple	As above	No	Weak	Yes
9p23	TYRP1	No	A	0.86 (0.80, 0.93)	rs1408799	Not GW sig.	Yes	No	No
11q14.3	TYR	Yes	A	1.22 (1.14, 1.31)	rs1126809, rs1393350	1.30 (1.21, 1.39)	Yes	No	No
11q22.3	ATM	Yes	NA	NA	rs1801516	0.84 (0.79, 0.89)	No	No	Yes
11q13.3	CCND1	No	NA	NA	rs1485993	1.11 (1.04, 1.18)	No	No	Yes
12q13.11	VDR	No	C, OR <1.15	0.89 (0.82, 0.97)	rs1544410	Not GW sig.	No	No	Yes
15q13.1	OCA2	No	NA	NR	rs12913832	Not GW sig.	Yes	No	No
16q24.3	MC1R	Yes	A	1.83 (1.56, 2.15)	rs1805007	1.70 (1.54, 1.87)	Yes	No	Yes

20q11.22	*ASIP*	Yes	A	1.59 (1.41, 1.79)	**Multiple**	From ~1.20 to ~1.29	Yes	No	No
21q22.3	*MX2*	Yes	NA	NA	**rs45430**	0.88 (0.85, 0.92)	No	No	Yes
22q13.1	*PLA2G6*	No	NA	0.85 (0.79, 0.91)	**rs6001027**	0.85 (0.79, 0.91)	No	Yes	No

From: *J Invest Dermatol* (2012) 132:1763–1774. doi:10.1038/jid.2012.75; published online 5 Apr 2012

MelGene refers to the systematic review of Chatzinasiou et al. (2011), where the indicated quality scores and ORs were sourced from. Scores of A, B, and C refer to strong, moderate, and weak epidemiological evidence, respectively, as assessed by Chatzinasiou et al. (2011). Where a single candidate gene or associated SNP has been reliably associated at genome-wide significance levels, this has been indicated. Where available, the equivalent ORs from GWASs have been supplied for comparison with the systematic review ORs. If the likely mode of melanoma pathogenesis is via pigmentation, nevus proliferation, or others, this has been indicated

Abbreviations: *ASIP* agouti signaling protein, *ATM* ataxia telangiectasia mutated, *CASP8* caspase 8, *CCND1* cyclin D1, *CDKN2A* cyclin-dependent kinase inhibitor 2A, *GWAS* genome-wide association study, *HWE* Hardy–Weinberg equilibrium, *MC1R* melanocortin-1 receptor, *MTAP* methylthioadenosine phosphorylase, *MX2* homologues of myxovirus resistance 2, *NA* not applicable, *OCA2* oculocutaneous albinism type 2, *OR* odds ratio, *PARP1* poly (ADP-ribose) polymerase 1, *PLA2G6* phospholipase A2, group VI, *sig.* significant, *SLC45A2* solute carrier family 45 member 2, *SNP* single-nucleotide polymorphism, *TERT* telomerase reverse transcriptase, *TYR* tyrosinase, *TYRP1* TYR-related protein 1, *VDR* vitamin D receptor

Biochemical and Serological Markers

- Please see table:

Tumor type	Marker	Recommended use	Recommending organizations
Melanoma	TA90-IC	Monitoring, prognosis	ACS, NACB
	S-100, HMB45 (gp100)	Diagnosis, usually used in combination	ACS, NACB
	S-100B (serum)	Monitoring, prognosis	ACS, NACB
	c-Kit	Response to tyrosine kinase inhibitors (TKI)	ACS

ACS American Cancer Society, *NACB* National Academy of Clinical Biochemistry

Past Medical History

- Having more than 50 ordinary moles on the body increases the risk of developing melanoma.
- Having dysplastic nevi increases the risk of developing melanoma.
- People with weakened immune systems have an increased risk of developing melanoma including people with HIV/AIDS and those who have had organ transplants.
- People with a past history of melanoma are at an approximately 100-fold increased risk for developing a second primary tumor some time after the original occurrence.
- At least 5 % of persons who have had 1 melanoma will develop a subsequent, independent melanoma.

Family History

- About 10 % of all people with melanoma have a family history of melanoma.
- If there is a family history of melanoma in one or more of first-degree relatives (parent, brother or sister, or child), the risk of developing melanoma is higher.
- Depending on the number of affected relatives, the risk can be up to eight times greater than that in the general population.

Comorbidities

- People with the following conditions are at higher risk for developing melanoma:

  - Xeroderma pigmentosum
  - Numerous actinic keratoses
  - Lentigines

Age/Gender/Ethnicity/Nutrition/Lifestyle

- Having fair skin and less pigment (melanin), blond or red hair, light-colored eyes, and freckles increases the risk of developing melanoma.

- A history of 1 or more severe, blistering sunburns as a child or teenager can increase the risk of developing melanoma as an adult.
- Exposure to UV radiation (from the sun and/or tanning beds) increases the risk of developing melanoma and other skin cancers.
- People living closer to the earth's equator are at increased risk for developing melanoma.
- People living at high altitude are at increased risk for developing melanoma.

Recommendations

- Identify and report abnormal nevi as early as possible, using the following guidelines:

   A. Asymmetry: one-half different from the other
   B. Border: irregular, scalloped, or poorly defined
   C. Color: varying from one area to another (shades of tan and brown; black; sometimes white, red, or blue)
   D. Diameter: usually greater than 6 mm in diameter but it can be smaller
   E. Evolving: a mole (even small) that is changing in color, aspect, and size or starts to itch or bleeds

- Evaluate/avoid/attenuate risk factors, if possible. Please see above and the table:

Risk factors	Estimated relative risk[a]
New mole, preexisting mole that has changed or is changing	High (10–400)[b]
Dysplastic nevi, prior melanoma, and familial melanoma	500
Dysplastic nevi, no prior melanoma, and familial melanoma	148
Dysplastic nevi, no personal or family history of melanoma	7–27
Congenital nevus	2–21
20 nevi at least 2 mm in diameter (if 50 nevi or more)	7–14 (then 54)
5 nevi—7 mm in diameter (if 8 nevi)	6 (then 17)
5 mol at least 5 mm in diameter (if 12 nevi or more)	10 (then 41)
Lentigo maligna	10
Caucasian (vs. African American)	20
Prior cutaneous melanoma	9
Cutaneous melanoma in first-degree blood relative	8
Immunosuppression	4
Sun-induced freckles by history	3
Sun sensitivity, relative inability to tan	3
Red hair, blond hair, or green or blue eyes	1–2
Excessive sun exposure	?

From: *Fitzpatrick's Dermatol Gen Med*, p 1026, Table 90.1
[a]Degree of increased risk for people with the risk factor compared to people without the risk factor. Data derived from case-control and prospective studies. Relative risk of 1.0 indicates no increased risk
[b]Risk estimated to be increased 10-fold to 400-fold, depending on the prevalence of new or changing mole in the general population

1.18.1.2   Preventive Advice

Chemical

- Vitamin D may help to prevent melanoma.
- Folic acid (or vitamin B9) protects cells from cancer.

Lifestyle

- Avoid the sun between about 10 am and 4 pm
- Wear sunscreen all year long. Choose a broad-spectrum sunscreen that has a sun protection factor (SPF) of at least 15. Use a generous amount of sunscreen on all exposed skin, including the lips, tips of the ears, back of the hands, and neck. Apply sunscreen 20–30 min before sun exposure and reapply it frequently while exposed to the sun. Reapply it after swimming or exercising.
- Wear protective tightly woven clothing that covers the arms and legs.
- Wear a broad-brimmed hat.
- Wear sunglasses. Look for those that block both types of UV radiation: UVA and UVB rays.
- Avoid tanning beds.
- Examine the skin regularly for changes. With the help of mirrors, check the face, neck, ears, scalp, chest and trunk, and the tops and undersides of the arms and hands. Examine both the front and back of the legs and feet, including the soles and the spaces between toes. Also check the genital area and between the buttocks. Report any changes to a physician.
- Have skin regularly examined by a physician.

Nutrition

- Foods containing vitamin D (dairies) may help to prevent melanoma.
- Foods containing folic acid are useful (e.g., cowpeas, chickpeas, beans, lentils). Please use the following link: http://folicacidnow.net/folic_acid/food_chart.shtml.

1.19   Multiple Sclerosis

1.19.1   Risk Assessment and Prevention of Multiple Sclerosis (MS)

1.19.1.1   Risk Assessment

Genetic Markers

- Traditional linkage scans have identified only one risk haplotype for MS (at HLA on chromosome 6), which explains only a fraction of the increased risk to siblings.

- Genetic linkage to the major histocompatibility complex (MHC) on chromosome 6 can be explained by the HLA-DR2 allelic association.
- Alleles of the MHC defined as DR15 and DEQ6 are associated with an increased risk of developing MS.
- The MHC explains between 17 and 62 % of the genetic etiology of MS.
- DR17 increases the risk of developing MS.
- Sporadic and familial MS share a common genetic susceptibility.
- Please see Table 1.40 for top non-MHC GWA and validation results for MS.

Biochemical and Serological Markers

- Anti-Epstein–Barr virus nuclear antigen 1 (anti-EBNA-1) antibody titers are risk factors for developing MS, independently from the DR15 allele.
- Carriers of the DR15 allele with elevated anti-EBNA-1 antibody titers may have a markedly increased risk of MS.
- Many biomarkers have been studied in the following categories:

  - Reflecting alteration of the immune system
  - Showing axonal/neuronal damage
  - Evidencing blood-brain barrier disruption
  - Displaying demyelination
  - Witnessing oxidative stress and excitotoxicity
  - Illustrating gliosis
  - Indicating remyelination and repair

Past Medical History

- A variety of viruses have been linked to MS.
- Infection with the Epstein–Barr virus results in a higher risk of developing MS.

Family History

- The risk of developing MS for first-degree relatives is increased some 20-fold over the general population.
- Twin studies have shown monozygotic concordance rates of 25–30 % compared to 4 % for dizygotic twins and siblings.
- Studies of adoptees and half sibs show that familial risk is determined by genes, but environmental factors strongly influence observed geographic differences.

Comorbidities

- Autoimmune thyroid disease increases the risk of developing MS.
- Type 1 diabetes increases the risk of developing MS.
- Inflammatory bowel disease increases the risk of developing MS.

Table 1.40 Top non-MHC GWA screen and validation results for multiple sclerosis

Gene (NCBI ID)	Chromosomal position	Biological function(s)	GWA screen Family[a]	Validation Case control[b]	Combined[c]	Overall Combined[d]	Odds ratio
IL-2RA, interleukin 2 receptor, alpha (3559)	**10p15**	Apoptosis, immune response	1×10^{-3}	1×10^{-3}	5×10^{-4}	3×10^{-8}	1.25
IL-7R, interleukin 7 receptor (16197)	**5p13**	Cell survival, immune response	6×10^{-3}	2×10^{-2}	3×10^{-5}	3×10^{-7}	1.18
CLEC16A, C-type lectin domain family 16, A (23274)	**16p13**	Sugar-binding, C-type lectin	3×10^{-2}	7×10^{-3}	2×10^{-5}	4×10^{-6}	1.14
RPL5, ribosomal protein L5 (6125)	**1p22**	Ribosomal protein, chaperone for the 5S rRNA	4×10^{-4}	2×10^{-4}	9×10^{-4}	8×10^{-6}	1.15
DBC1, deleted in bladder cancer 1 (1620)	**9q33**	Cell cycle arrest, apoptosis	1×10^{-4}	2×10^{-4}	1×10^{-3}	8×10^{-6}	1.17
CD58, lymphocyte function-associated antigen 3 (965)	**1p13**	Cell–cell adhesion, immune response	1×10^{-3}	3×10^{-5}	2×10^{-3}	2×10^{-5}	1.24
ALK, anaplastic lymphoma receptor tyrosine kinase (238)	**2p23**	Tyrosine kinase receptor, brain development	1×10^{-4}	1×10^{-2}	3×10^{-3}	7×10^{-5}	1.37
FAM69A, family with sequence similarity 69, A (388650)	**1p22**	Protein binding	2×10^{-5}	2×10^{-2}	2×10^{-3}	9×10^{-5}	1.12

From: *Nat Rev Genet* (2008) 9:516–526. doi:10.1038/nrg2395
Listed are the eight non-MHC SNPs showing the highest statistical evidence of association after replication as reported by the International Multiple Sclerosis Genetics Consortium.
GWA genome-wide association, *MHC* major histocompatibility complex, *MS* multiple sclerosis, *NCBI* National Center for Biotechnology Information
[a]931 MS trios
[b]931 cases, 2,431 controls
[c]609 MS trios, 2,322 MS cases, 2,987 controls
[d]1,540 MS trios, 2,322 MS cases, 5,418 controls

Similarly:

- Female MS patients have an increased risk of developing breast cancer.
- MS patients have a higher risk of developing primary brain tumors.
- Patients with MS have an increased risk of developing urinary organ cancer.
- Researchers found a 78 % decreased risk of cancer (except the ones mentioned above) among MS patients, which may be due to a healthier lifestyle.

Age/Gender/Ethnicity/Nutrition/Lifestyle

- MS most commonly affects people between 20 and 40 years old.
- Women are about twice as likely as men to develop MS.
- Caucasians particularly those whose families originated in Northern Europe are at highest risk for developing MS.
- People of Asian, African, or Native American descent have the lowest risk of developing MS.
- MS is far more common in Europe, southern Canada, northern United States, New Zealand, and southeastern Australia.
- The risk of developing MS seems to increase with latitude.
- A child who moves from a high-risk area to a low-risk area, or vice versa, tends to have the risk level associated with his or her new home area. However, if the move occurs after puberty, he/she usually retains the risk level associated with his or her first home.
- One cause of multiple sclerosis is heavy metals, usually mercury from fish, dental amalgam, or other sources. Other heavy metals and even some chemicals (e.g., pesticides) can cause MS.

Recommendations

- Eliminate/avoid/attenuate risk factors, if possible (please see above and below), in particular exposure to chemicals and contact with heavy metals.
- Avoid immune system deregulating and suppressing agents.

1.19.1.2 Preventive Advice

Chemical

- Linoleic acid seems to prevent MS.
- Vitamin D is associated with a lower incidence of MS.
- Omega-3 fatty acids may be helpful.

Lifestyle

- Get regular exercise (please see Sect. 2.1).
- Reduce stress (please see Sect. 2.2).
- Do not smoke/quit smoking or chewing tobacco (please see Sect. 2.3).

Nutrition

- Antioxidant foods such as berries, oranges, spinach, and carrots can be beneficial.
- Caffeine, green tea, and tart cherries may all help ward off MS.
- Resveratrol (found, e.g., in red wine) has shown some promise in the prevention of MS.

1.20   Myocardial Infarction

1.20.1   Risk Assessment and Prevention of Myocardial Infarction (MI)

1.20.1.1   Risk Assessment

Genetic Markers

- On chromosomes 3 and 12, scientists suspect that 2 genes are associated with the risk of developing MI: (1) the MRAS gene plays an important role in cardiovascular biology and (2) the HNF1A gene is closely associated with cholesterol metabolism.
- On chromosome 6, the LPA gene regulates the concentration of a specific lipoprotein Lp(a).
- Three genes associated with an increased risk of developing MI can be found on chromosomes 2, 6, and 21.
- Variants at the 9p21 locus are associated with the risk of developing MI. This association represents one of the most consistent and robust SNP disease associations in the GWAS era, having been replicated in several independent samples in numerous ethnicities.
- There are many genetic markers of MI as shown in Table 1.41.

Biochemical and Serological Markers

- High LDL cholesterol and/or triglyceride levels as well as low levels of HDL cholesterol increase the risk of MI.
- There are more than 44 biomarkers associated with the risk of developing MI in particular in the following categories: lipid, inflammatory, hemostatic, endothelial, and adipocyte hormones. Please see Table 1.42.

Table 1.41 Loci associated with MI

Locus	Nearest gene	Risk allele frequency	p	Relative risk for MI
q22.3	MRAS	0.15	7×10^{-13}	1.15 (1.11–1.19)
12q24.31	HNF1A	0.36	5×10^{-7}	1.08 (1.05–1.11)
9p21.3	CDKN2A, CDKN2B	0.56	3×10^{-44}	1.29 (1.25–1.34)
1p13.3	CELSR2, PSRC1, SORT1	0.81	8×10^{-12}	1.19 (1.13–1.26)
21q22.11	SLC5A3, MRPS6, KCNE2	0.13	6×10^{-11}	1.20 (1.14–1.27)
1q41	MIA3	0.72	1×10^{-9}	1.14 (1.10–1.19)
6p24.1	PHACTR1	0.65	1×10^{-9}	1.12 (1.08–1.17)
19p13.2	LDLR	0.75	2×10^{-9}	1.15 (1.10–1.20)
10q11.21	CXCL12	0.84	7×10^{-9}	1.17 (1.11–1.24)
1p32.3	PCSK9	0.81	1×10^{-8}	1.15 (1.10–1.21)
2q33.1	WDR12	0.14	1×10^{-8}	1.17 (1.11–1.23)
6q25.3	SLC22A3,LPAL2,LPA	0.02	4×10^{-15}	1.82 (1.57–2.12)
6q25.3	SLC22A3,LPAL2,LPA	0.16	1×10^{-9}	1.20 (1.13–1.28)
12q24.12	SH2B3	0.38	9×10^{-8}	1.13 (1.08–1.18)

From: *Circulation* (2010) 122(22): 2323–2334
Loci were selected from the GWAS catalog on the basis of a search for the following phenotypes
Coronary disease, CAD, major CVD, MI, and MI (early onset). We also included the 12q24.12
locus, which has been associated with eosinophil levels, asthma, and MI

Table 1.42 Biomarkers for identifying an MI-vulnerable patient

Biomarker	Methodology standardized	Methodology available/convenient	Linked to disease prospectively	Additive to FHS risk score	Tracks with disease treatment
Arterial vulnerability					
Serological biomarkers of arterial vulnerability					
Abnormal lipid profile	+++	+++	+++	Part of score	+++
Apo B	+	+	+++	+	+
Lp(a)	+/−	+	+++	−	?
LDL particle No.	+/−	−	+	−	?
CETP	+/−	+/−	+	?	?
Lp-PLA2	−	−	+	?	?
Inflammation					
Hs-CRP	+++	+++	+++	+	+/?
sICAM-1	+/−	+/−	++	?	?
IL-6	−	−	++	?	?
IL-18	−	−	++	?	?
SAA	−	−	−	?	?

(continued)

Table 1.42 (continued)

Biomarker	Methodology standardized	Methodology available/convenient	Linked to disease prospectively	Additive to FHS risk score	Tracks with disease treatment
MPO	+	−	+	?	−
sCD40	?	−	+	?	?
Oxidized LDL	−	+	+	?	?
GPX1 activity	−	−	+	?	?
Nitrotyrosine	−	−	+	+/?	+
Homocysteine	+++	+++	+++	?	?
Cystatin C	+	−	+	?	?
Natriuretic peptides	+	++	+++	?	+
ADMA	+	−	++	?	?
MMP-9	−	−	+	?	?
TIMP-1	+	−	+	?	?
Structural markers of arterial vulnerability					
Carotid IMT	++	+/?	++	+/?	+
Coronary artery calcium	+++	+	+	+/?	?
Functional markers of arterial vulnerability					
Blood pressure	+++	++	+++	Part of score	+++
Endothelial dysfunction	+	++	?	+	
Arterial stiffness	++	++	+	?	+
Ankle–brachial index	+++	+++	++	+/?	?
Urine albumin excretion	++	++	++	+/?	++
Blood vulnerability					
Serological markers of blood vulnerability					
Hypercoagulable					
Fibrinogen	++	++	+++	?	?
D-Dimer	+	+	++	?	?
Decreased fibrinolysis					
TPA/PAI-1	+/−	+	++	?	?
Increased coagulation factors					

Table 1.42   (continued)

Biomarker	Methodology standardized	Methodology available/convenient	Linked to disease prospectively	Additive to FHS risk score	Tracks with disease treatment
von Willebrand factor	++	++	+	?	?
Myocardial vulnerability					
Structural markers of myocardial vulnerability					
LVH, LV dysfunction	++	++	++	?	++
Functional markers of myocardial vulnerability					
Exercise stress test/stress echo	++	++	++	++	++
PET	++	–	–	?	?
Serological markers of myocardial vulnerability					
Troponins	++	++	++	?	?

From: *Circulation* (2006) 113(19):2335–2362
FHS Framingham Heart Study, *– no*, ? unknown or questionable/equivocal data, + some evidence, ++ good evidence, +++ strong evidence, *ADMA* asymmetrical dimethylarginine, *Apo B* apolipoprotein B, *CETP* cholesterol ester transfer protein, *GPX1* glutathione peroxidase, *IL* interleukin, *IMT* intimal–medial thickness, *Lp(a)* lipoprotein a, *LpPLA2* lipoprotein-associated phospholipase A2, *LV* left ventricle, *LVH* LV hypertrophy, *MMP* matrix metalloproteinase, *MPO* myeloperoxidase, *SAA* serum amyloid A, *sCD40L* soluble CD40 ligand, *sICAM* soluble intercellular adhesion molecule, *PAI-1* plasminogen activator inhibitor 1, *PET* positron emission tomography, *TIMP* tissue inhibitor of matrix metalloproteinases, and *TPA* tissue plasminogen activator

Past Medical History

- Anyone with heart disease (previous heart attack or stroke, past or present angina pain, evidence of vascular disease, or abdominal aortic aneurysm) has more than a 20 % chance of a heart attack in the next 10 years.
- A history of preeclampsia increases the lifetime risk of MI.

Family History

- If siblings, parents, or grandparents have had heart attacks, it increases the risk of MI. The overall odds ratio (OR) for those having ≥1 first-degree relatives with ischemic heart disease is 2.1 and 3.8 for ≥2 relatives. The ORs for all those with an affected parent or sibling are similar.

- A genetic condition that raises cholesterol levels and/or blood pressure in a family increases the risk of heart attack.

Comorbidities

- Diabetes greatly increases the risk of MI.
- High blood pressure increases the risk of MI.
- Metabolic syndrome increases the risk of MI.
- Small vessel disease, also known as coronary microvascular disease, increases the risk of MI.
- Coronary artery disease increases the risk of MI.
- Kawasaki disease increases the risk of MI.
- Left ventricular hypertrophy increases the risk of MI.
- Obesity increases the risk of MI.

Age/Gender/Ethnicity/Nutrition/Lifestyle

- Men who are 45 or older and women who are 55 or older are more likely to have an MI than younger men and women.
- Smoking increases the risk of MI. It may cause 53 % of MIs among urban males in India.
- Lack of exercise increases the risk of MI.
- Stress increases the risk of MI.
- Using cocaine or amphetamines increases the risk of MI.
- There is concern that vitamin D supplements may increase the risk of MI.

Recommendations

- Eliminate/avoid/attenuate risk factors, if possible (please see above and below).
- Calculate MI risk: http://hp2010.nhlbihin.net/atpiii/calculator.asp.

1.20.1.2   Preventive Advice

Chemical

- For people who are at risk or had an MI, physicians may prescribe the following drugs:

  - Aspirin or clopidogrel (Plavix®). However, these anticoagulants and ibuprofen (Advil®, Motrin®) or other NSAIDs increase the risk of gastrointestinal bleeding.
  - Beta-blockers.
  - Angiotensin-converting enzyme (ACE) inhibitors.

- Cholesterol-lowering medications such as statins, niacin, fibrates, and bile acid sequestrants.

• Vitamins C and E may reduce the risk of MI. They prevent LDL from adhering to the plaque.
• Do not take vitamin D, if not necessary.
• Magnesium decreases the risk of muscle spasm.
• Folic acid lowers the serum level of homocysteine.

Lifestyle

• Exercise regularly (please see Sect. 2.1).
• Lose weight, if necessary, by increasing caloric output (exercising) and decreasing caloric intake (dieting).
• Reduce stress (please see Sect. 2.2).
• Do not smoke/stop smoking or chewing tobacco (please see Sect. 2.3).
• Control blood pressure.
• Have regular medical checkups.

Nutrition

• Drink red wine, if there is no contraindication (e.g., alcoholism or liver condition). Please see Sect. 2.4.
• Follow a cholesterol-lowering diet. The Stanford University Health Improvement Program recommends the Mediterranean diet. Please also see Sect. 2.7.

1.21 Obesity

1.21.1 Risk Assessment and Prevention of Obesity

1.21.1.1 Risk Assessment

Genetic Markers

• Obesity is a complex multifactorial chronic condition that develops from an intricate interaction of genetic factors with the environment. The list of genes and genetic markers associated with human obesity has increased in recent years, for example:

  - 8 variants show individual associations with childhood BMI in/near FTO, MC4R, TMEM18, GNPDA2, KCTD15, NEGR1, BDNF, and ETV5.
  - People with 2 copies of the FTO gene (fat mass- and obesity-associated gene) weigh 3–4 kg more and have a 1.67-fold greater risk of obesity compared to those without the risk allele.

Table 1.43 Selected genes with variants that have been associated with obesity

Gene symbol	Gene name	Gene product's role in energy balance
ADIPOQ	Adipocyte-, C1q-, and collagen domain-containing	Produced by fat cells, adiponectin promotes energy expenditure
FTO	Fat mass- and obesity-associated gene	Promotes food intake
LEP	Leptin	Produced by fat cells
LEPR	Leptin receptor	When bound by leptin, inhibits appetite
INSIG2	Insulin-induced gene 2	Regulation of cholesterol and fatty acid synthesis
MC4R	Melanocortin 4 receptor	When bound by alpha-melanocyte-stimulating hormone, stimulates appetite
PCSK1	Proprotein convertase subtilisin/kexin type 1	Regulates insulin biosynthesis
PPARG	Peroxisome proliferator-activated receptor gamma	Stimulates lipid uptake and development of fat tissue

From the Centers for Disease Control and Prevention: http://www.cdc.gov/genomics/resources/diseases/obesity/obesedit.htm

- – The Lewis phenotype Le(a-b-) is a genetic marker of obesity.
- – APOA-IV gene polymorphisms are associated with obesity-related traits.

- • The obesity gene map shows putative loci on all chromosomes except Y.
- • Please see Table 1.43 for selected genes with variants that have been associated with obesity.

Biochemical and Serological Markers

- • Insulin, leptin, resistin, interleukin-6 (IL-6), insulin-like growth factor 1 (IGF-1), tumor necrosis factor-alpha (TNF-alpha), adiponectin, hs-C-reactive protein (CRP), glutathione peroxidase, and isoprostane have been used as biomarkers of obesity.

Past Medical History

- • Some diseases can cause obesity such as:

  - – Prader–Willi syndrome
  - – Cushing's syndrome
  - – Polycystic ovary syndrome

- • Some medical problems, such as arthritis, may result in and from weight gain.
- • Some medicines such as insulin, sulfonylureas, thiazolidinediones, atypical antipsychotics, antidepressants, steroids, certain anticonvulsants (phenytoin and valproate), pizotifen, some forms of hormonal contraception, antidepressants, and antipsychotics can induce weight gain and obesity.

- Quitting smoking can induce weight gain and obesity. Most people who quit smoking gain 4–10 lb in the first 6 months after quitting. Some people gain as much as 25–30 lb.
- For women, menopause can lead to weight gain and obesity.
- Some women do not lose the weight they gained during pregnancy.

Family History

- Obesity tends to run in families not only because of genetics but also because family members tend to have similar eating, lifestyle, and activity habits.
- If one or both parents are obese, the risk for children to develop obesity is increased.

Comorbidities

- Hypothyroidism rarely causes obesity.

Similarly:

The following diseases/conditions are associated with obesity:
- Skin diseases (cellulitis, candidiasis, dermatophytoses)
- Sleep apnea
- Pickwickian syndrome
- Hypertension
- Joint disorders (arthritis in the knees, and/or ankles, ligament tears, etc.)
- Cardiovascular disorders (congestive heart failure, myocardial infarction, stroke, etc.)
- Renal disorders such as chronic renal failure
- Type II diabetes mellitus
- Hyperlipidemia (hypercholesterolemia and elevated triglycerides)
- Psychosocial disability
- Metabolic syndrome
- Fatty liver disease
- Urinary incontinence
- Erectile dysfunction
- Lymphedema
- Cancers:

  – Men: colon, rectum, prostate
  – Women: uterus, biliary tract, breast, ovary

- Thromboembolic disorders
- Digestive tract disorders (such as gallstones, gastroesophageal reflux disease, diaphragmatic hernia)
- Increased surgical and obstetrical risks. Other increased risks include:

  – Pulmonary functional impairment
  – Endocrine abnormalities
  – Increased hemoglobin concentration

Age/Gender/Ethnicity/Nutrition/Lifestyle

- The risk of developing obesity increases with age.
- Certain social and economic issues may be linked to obesity such as not having safe areas to exercise, not having been taught healthy ways of cooking, or not having money to buy healthy foods.
- People are more likely to become obese if their friends are obese.
- Sedentarity increases the risk of developing obesity.
- High-calorie diet and drinks, fast food, skipping breakfast, and eating oversized portions contribute to weight gain.
- The risk of obesity soars with family income in some countries.
- In the United States, poorer people have an increased prevalence of obesity.
- Drinking alcohol may induce weight gain and obesity.
- Stress, anxiety, depression, or not sleeping well can induce weight gain and obesity.

Recommendations

- Eliminate/avoid/attenuate risk factors, if possible (please see above and below).
- Eliminate medical causes (please see above).
- Calculate BMI (please see below).

English formula
BMI = weight in pounds/(height in inches × height in inches) × 703
Metric formula
BMI = weight in kilograms/(height in meters × height in meters)

BMI	*Weight status*
Below 18.5	Underweight
18.5–24.9	Normal
25.0–29.9	Overweight
30.0 and higher	Obese
40.0 and higher	Extremely obese

- Kids fall into one of four categories:

  1. Underweight: BMI below the 5th percentile
  2. Normal weight: BMI at the 5th and less than the 85th percentile
  3. Overweight: BMI at the 85th and below 95th percentiles
  4. Obese: BMI at or above 95th percentile

1.21.1.2 Preventive Advice

Chemical

- The following supplements may help to prevent obesity:

  – Vitamin B2
  – Vitamin B3

- Vitamin B5
- Vitamin B6
- Vitamin C

As well as:

- Choline
- Inositol

Lifestyle

Prevent obesity by:

- Monitoring weight.
- Getting regular exercise (please see Sect. 2.1).
- Reducing stress (please see Sect. 2.2).
- Sleeping well (please see Sect. 2.2).
- Losing weight by increasing caloric output through exercise (please see Sect. 2.1) and decreasing caloric intake (please see below). Losing weight is a family affair.

Nutrition

- Reduce caloric intake by downsizing portions using a balanced diet (e.g., Nutrisystem*) and reduce cholesterol and fat in diet (please see Sect. 2.7). The Stanford University Health Improvement Program recommends the Mediterranean diet for cholesterol control.
- Be consistent. Maintain a healthy diet all year long.
- Drink alcohol with moderation (please see Sect. 2.4).

1.22   Osteoarthritis

1.22.1   Risk Assessment and Prevention of Osteoarthritis (OA)

1.22.1.1   Risk Assessment

Genetic Markers

- Candidate gene and genome-wide linkage studies have identified genes in the bone morphogenetic pathway (e.g., GDF5), the thyroid regulation pathway (DIO2), and apoptotic pathways involved in genetic risk of large joint OA.
- Genome-wide association studies have reported structural genes (COL6A4/ DVWA), inflammation-related genes (PTGS2/PLA2G4A), and a locus on

chr 7q22 as well as a gene involved in transcriptional regulation (A2BP1) that are associated with knee OA.

- Genetic influence ranges from 39 to 65 % in the development of hand and knee OA.
- Certain gene mutations have been linked only to a particular site of OA (e.g., knee, hip, or hand) implying that each site might have its own genetic basis.
- Please see table in *Nat Rev Rheumatol* (2012) 8:77–89, via the following link:

  http://www.nature.com/nrrheum/journal/v8/n2/full/nrrheum.2011.199.html.

Biochemical and Serological Markers

- In the table below, the BIPED scheme (burden of disease, investigative, prognostic, efficacy of intervention and diagnostic) is used for the classification of OA markers, as proposed by Bauer et al. in 2006, to describe the potential uses of a given marker.

Medscape®	www.medscape.com			
Tissue	Molecule	Markers of synthesis	Markers of degradation	BIPED classification
Bone	Type I collagen		PYD[a]	B
			NTX-I[a,b]	D
			CTX-I[a,b]	P
	Noncollagenous proteins	Osteocalcin[b]		P
Cartilage	Type II collagen	PIIANP[b]		P
		Total PIINP		D
		PIICP[b,c]		D P
			CTX-II[a,c]	D B P E
			HELIX-II[a]	P
			Coll 2-1[a,b]	P
			Coll 2–1 NO$_2$[a,b]	P
			C2C[a,b]	P E
			C1,2C[a,b]	P E
	Aggrecan	Epitope 846 (cartilage content[c])		E
	Nonaggrecan and noncollagenous proteins		COMP[b,c]	D B P
			Pentosidine[a,b]	P
	Proteases and their inhibitors		MMPs[b]	B P E
			TIMPs[b]	B P

Medscape®	www.medscape.com			
Tissue	Molecule	Markers of synthesis	Markers of degradation	BIPED classification
Synovium	Type III collagen		Glo–Gal–PYD[a]	E
	Noncollagenous	YKL-40[b,c]		B E
	proteins	Hyaluronic acid[b]		B P

Source: *Nat Clin Pract Rheumatol* ©2007 Nature Publishing Group

Abbreviations: BIPED classification, *B* burden of disease, *I* inveetigative, *P* prognostic, *E* efficacy of intervention, *D* diagnostic, *C1,2C* assay that detects COL2-2/4C (ahort) epitope, *C2C* assay that detects COL2-2/4 C (long) epitope, *Coll 2-1* nine-amino-acid peptide of type II collagen, Coll 2-1 NO$_2$, nitrated form of Coll 2-1, *COMP* cartilage oligomeric protein, *CTX-1* C-terminal cross-linked telopeptide of type I collagen, *CTX-II* C-terminal cross-linked telopeptide of type II collagen, *Glc–Gal–PYD* glucosyl–galactosyl–pyridinoline, *HELIX-II* helical type II collagen, *MMP* matrix metalloproteinase, *NTX-I* N-terminal cross-linked telopeptide of type I collagen, *PIIANP* N-propeptide IIA of collagen type II, *PIICP* C-propeptide of collagen type II, *PIINP* N-propeptide II of collagen type II, *PYD* pyridinoline, *TIMP* tissue inhibitor of matrix metalloproteinase, *YKL-40* cartilage glycoprotein 39

[a]Urine
[b]Serum
[c]Synovial fluid

Past Medical History

- People born with malformed joints or defective cartilage have an increased risk of developing OA.

Family History

- People who have relatives with OA are at increased risk for developing the disease.
- An identical twin has a twofold higher chance of developing OA of the hand or knee if the other twin has the same disease.
- Sisters of women with hand OA have a twofold increased risk of developing the disease compared to the general population. This risk is increased by five- to sevenfold if the sibling has a severe form of the disease.

Comorbidities

- People with bleeding disorders such as hemophilia are at increased risk for developing OA.
- People with disorders that block the blood supply near a joint and lead to avascular necrosis are at increased risk for developing OA.
- People with other types of arthritis, such as chronic gout, pseudogout (chondrocalcinosis), Charcot's joints, and rheumatoid arthritis, are at increased risk for developing OA.

- People with diabetes are at increased risk for developing OA.
- People with inflammatory diseases such as Perthes disease or with Lyme disease are at increased risk for developing OA.
- People with septic arthritis are at increased risk for developing OA.
- People with poor ligaments are at increased risk for developing OA.
- People with Marfan syndrome are at increased risk for developing OA.
- People with alkaptonuria are at increased risk for developing OA.
- People with hemochromatosis and Wilson's disease are at increased risk for developing OA.
- People with Ehlers–Danlos syndrome are at increased risk for developing OA.
- Obese people carry more body weight, which places more stress on weight-bearing joints, such as the knees. Therefore, they have an increased risk of developing OA.

Age/Gender/Ethnicity/Nutrition/Lifestyle

- The risk of developing OA increases with age.
- Before age 55, OA occurs equally in men and women. After age 55, it is more common in women.
- Caucasians and African Americans have an overall higher risk of developing osteoarthritis than other racial and ethnic groups.
- Injuries from sports, accident, or surgery may increase the risk of developing OA.
- Sedentary lifestyle increases the risk of developing OA.
- Repetitive stress on a particular joint on a job, for example, predisposes that joint to developing OA.

Recommendations

- Eliminate/avoid/attenuate risk factors, if possible (please see above and below).

1.22.1.2   Preventive Advice

Chemical

- Glucosamine may help maintain joint health and reduce the risk of developing degenerative joint disease, in particular OA.
- Chondroitin may be helpful in preventing OA.
- Bromelain, an enzyme derived from the stem of the pineapple fruit, may reduce inflammation and the risk of developing osteoarthritis.
- Omega-3 fatty acids may reduce inflammation and the risk of developing osteoarthritis.

Note: Supplements may cause side effects and interact with drugs.

Lifestyle

- Get regular exercise (please see Sect. 2.1).
- Control weight and maintain a healthy weight.
- Avoid repetitive stress and injuries on joints.
- Avoid single joint injury.
- Avoid unnatural and awkward motions.
- Listen to your pain and do not exercise through it. Consider it a stop sign.
- Good posture and proper body mechanics are important.
- Try acupuncture.
- Try tai chi.
- Try yoga.

Nutrition

- Eat a balanced diet. The Stanford University Health Improvement Program recommends the Mediterranean diet.
- Garlic, watercress, parsley, celery, and cold-water fish can be beneficially included into the diet.
- Herbal supplements including ginger and turmeric may also prevent inflammation and osteoarthritis.

1.23 Prostate Cancer

1.23.1 Risk Assessment and Prevention of Prostate Cancer

1.23.1.1 Risk Assessment

Genetic Markers

- Mutations on BRCA1 and BRCA2 genes increase the risk of developing prostate cancer.
- Multiple chromosome alterations are linked to an increased risk of prostate cancer, for example, on chromosomes 3, 6, 7, 10, 11, 19, and X.
- Multiple regions within the 8q24 chromosome independently affect the risk for prostate cancer.
- 5 single-nucleotide polymorphisms located at chromosomal loci 8q and 17q (rs1859962, rs6983267, rs4430796, rs1447295, and rs16901979) were found to have a cumulative increased association with prostate cancer in multiple studies.
- The population-attributable risk of the locus marked by rs6983267 is higher than the locus marked by rs1447295 (21 % vs. 9 %).

- Black men are more likely to carry risk-associated SNPs than high-risk Caucasian men.
- 2 variants on chromosome 17 are associated with prostate cancer. They are 33 Mb apart. The risks conferred by these variants are moderate individually (allele odds ratio of about 1.20), but because they are common, their joint population-attributable risk is substantial. One of the variants is in TCF2 (HNF1β).
- Please see Table 1.44 for proposed prostate cancer susceptibility loci.

Biochemical and Serological Markers

- Elevated levels of luteinizing hormone and of testosterone/dihydrotestosterone ratios are associated with mildly increased risks of prostate cancer.

Table 1.44 Proposed prostate cancer susceptibility loci

Gene	Location	Candidate gene	Clinical testing	Proposed phenotype	Comments
HPC1/RNASEL (OMIM)	1q25	*RNASEL*	Not available	Younger age at prostate cancer diagnosis (<65 years) Higher tumor grade (Gleason score)	Evidence of linkage is strongest in families with at least five affected persons, young age at diagnosis, and male-to-male transmission
				More advanced stage at diagnosis	*RNASEL* mutations have been identified in a few 1q-linked families.
PCAP (OMIM)	1q42.2–43	None	Not available	Younger age at prostate cancer diagnosis (<65 years) and more aggressive disease	Evidence of linkage is strongest in European families
HPCX (OMIM)	Xq27–28	None	Not available	Unknown	May explain observation that an unaffected man with an affected brother has a higher risk than an unaffected man with an affected father

Table 1.44 (continued)

Gene	Location	Candidate gene	Clinical testing	Proposed phenotype	Comments
CAPB (OMIM)	1p36	None	Not available	Younger age at prostate cancer diagnosis (<65 years) One or more cases of brain cancer	Strongest evidence of linkage was initially described in families with both prostate and brain cancer; follow-up studies indicate that this locus may be associated specifically with early-onset prostate cancer but not necessarily with brain cancer
HPC20 (OMIM)	20q13	None	Not available	Later age at prostate cancer diagnosis No male-to-male transmission	Evidence of linkage is strongest in families with late age at diagnosis, fewer affected family members, and no male-to-male transmission
8p	8p21–23	MSR1	Not available	Unknown	In a genomic region commonly deleted in prostate cancer
8q	8q24	None	Not available	More aggressive disease	Data in some reports suggest that the population-attributable risk may be higher for African American men than for men of European origin

From: the National Cancer Institute

- A number of potential biomarkers have been identified that might provide additional predictive value in determining the risk of future prostate cancer. Please see Table 1.45.

- Other candidates include alpha-methylacyl coenzyme A racemase (AMACR or P5045), glutathione S-transferase P1 (GSTP1), chromogranin A (CGA, GRN-A), prostate-specific membrane antigen (PSMA), prostate stem cell antigen (PSCA), early prostate cancer antigen (EPCA), B7-H3, sacosine, caveolin-1, serum calcium, hypermethylation of PDLIM4 gene, PCA3/DD3, TMPRSS2-ERG gene fusion rearrangement, exosomes, Ki-67, GOLPH2, and DAB21P.
- For prostate-specific antigen (PSA), please see below in Recommendations.

Table 1.45 Description of the biological function of selected serum markers

Serum marker	Description/type	Biological function	Purpose
Chromogranin A	Prohormone peptide released by neuroendocrine cells	Uncertain definite function. Possesses calcium-binding abilities and may act through paracrine and autocrine manners	Prognosis
Neuron-specific enolase	Isomer of the glycolytic enzyme 2-phospho-D-glycerate hydrolase released by neuroendocrine cells	Uncertain definite function. Possibly serves as paracrine and autocrine factor	Prognosis
Human kallikrein 2	Serine protease with trypsin-like substrate specificity	Splits pro-PSA to create PSA	Diagnosis
Urokinase-type plasminogen activator system	Serine protease and transmembrane receptors	Converts plasminogen to plasmin	Diagnosis (fragments) and prognosis
Interleukin-6	Cytokine	Implicated in hematopoiesis and the immune response through mediation of B-cell differentiation and the acute-phase inflammatory response	Prognosis
Transforming growth factor-β	Cytokine	Involved in cellular proliferation, cellular chemotaxis, cellular differentiation, angiogenesis, humoral immunity, cell-mediated immunity, and wound healing	Prognosis
Prostate membrane-specific antigen	Type II integral membrane glycoprotein with cell surface carboxypeptidase function	Possesses folate hydrolase function. Also is involved in the cell stress reaction, signal transduction, cell migration, and nutrient uptake. May possess questionable receptor function	Diagnosis

Prostate-specific cell antigen	Glycosylphosphatidylinositol-anchored cell surface glycoprotein	Known cell surface marker. Perhaps involved in several stem cell activities involving proliferation or signal transduction	Prognosis
α-Methylacyl-CoA racemase (autoantibodies)	Peroxisomal and mitochondrial racemase	Engaged in bile acid synthesis, stereoisomerization, and β-oxidation of branched-chain fatty acids	Diagnosis
Early prostate cell antigen-1, antigen-2	Nuclear matrix protein	May be involved in early prostate carcinogenesis; however, has uncertain contribution to nuclear morphology	Diagnosis
GSTP1 hypermethylation	CpG island hypermethylation of DNA encoding the protein, glutathione S-transferase-π	Hypermethylation of GSTP1 inhibits transcription. GSTP1 usually acts by conjugation of oxidant and electrophilic carcinogens to glutathione to inactivate them	Diagnosis
Testosterone	Steroid hormone	Acts in the natural growth and support of the prostate gland and seminal vesicles. Many actions on sexual development and anabolism. Also involved in endocrine signal transduction	Prognosis

(continued)

Table 1.45 (continued)

Estrogen	Steroid hormone	Many effects on female sexual development. Also acts in the control of sperm development and in endocrine signal transduction	Prognosis
Sex hormone-binding globulin	Serum glycoprotein-binding protein	Adheres to and carries testosterone and estradiol. Also involved in endocrine signal transduction	Prognosis
Caveolin-1	Integral membrane protein	Works to regulate cholesterol metabolism and cellular transformation and is engaged in transducing cell-to-cell signals	Prognosis
E-Cadherin	Calcium-dependent cell adhesion protein	Plays major role as a cellular adhesion molecule in cell-to-cell adhesion of secretory tissues	Prognosis
β-Catenin	Adhesion protein (80 kDa fragment isolated in prostate cancer)	Aggregates with cadherin to regulate the formation of adherent junctions between cells	Prognosis
MMP-9	Zinc-dependent endogenous protease	Acts in cell migration through and degradation of the ECM and in cell–cell adhesion	Prognosis
Tissue inhibitor of MMPs (TIMP-1, TIMP-2)	Protease inhibitor	Prevents synthesis of ECM	Prognosis
Hepatocyte growth factor	Polypeptide growth factor (secretory protein of fibroblasts)	A cellular growth, motility, and morphogenic factor. Also, involved in cell scattering and angiogenesis	Diagnosis/prognosis

			Diagnosis/prognosis
MIC-1	Cytokine (TGF-β superfamily)	Uncertain role, but may induce apoptosis	
Cytokine macrophage MIF	Cytokine (secreted by lymphocytes)	Modulates inflammation and the immune response. Activates cellular proliferation and angiogenesis while inhibiting some tumor-suppressor genes	Diagnosis
hK11	Serine protease (human kallikrein superfamily)	Has an uncertain function. Acts like trypsin but, depending on the tissue or body compartment in which it is present, may possibly have many different functions	Diagnosis
Progastrin-releasing peptide (ProGRP 31-98)	Neuropeptide	Split to form GRP. GRP acts in the regulation of metabolism, behavior, smooth muscle activity, some exocrine and endocrine operations, and cellular chemotaxis.	Prognosis
Apolipoprotein A-II (8.9 kDa isoform)	Lipoprotein (abundant in HDL)	Affects plasma free fatty acid levels via operating in lipid metabolism and transport	Diagnosis
50.8 kDa protein	Unknown, identified by mass spectrometry	Uncertain function but possibly is parallel to the action of vitamin D-binding protein	Diagnosis
ILGF-1, ILGF-2	Growth hormone-dependent polypeptides	In the prostate gland, both modulate cellular proliferation, differentiation, and apoptosis. Also, acts in endocrine signal transduction	Diagnosis

(continued)

Table 1.45 (continued)

Leptin	Adipocyte-derived peptide	In metabolism, modulates hunger, energy use, and fat metabolism and is also known to induce angiogenesis	Diagnosis
Endoglin (CD105)	Homodimeric transmembrane glycoprotein	Controls TGF-β superfamily signaling pathway and therefore subsequently affects angiogenesis, cellular propagation, apoptosis, cell adhesion, and cell movement	Prognosis
EGFR family (c-erbB-1 (EGFR), c-erbB-2 (HER2/neu), c-erbB-3 (HER3), and c-erbB-4 (HER4))	Transmembrane glycoprotein receptors	Transduce signals for multiple growth factors	Diagnosis and prognosis
TSP-1	Homotrimeric extracellular matrix glycoprotein	Inhibits angiogenesis by inhibiting cell development, movement, and propagation and is also an effector molecule for the tumor-suppressor gene p53	Diagnosis
VEGF	Dimeric, heparin-binding protein	An important endothelial cell growth factor that controls angiogenesis and augments vascular permeability	Prognosis
Huntingtin-interacting protein 1 (autoantibodies)	Cytoplasmic clathrin-binding protein	Acts in growth factor receptor transport. Also, transforms fibroblasts by lengthening the half-life of growth factor receptors	Diagnosis

Prostasome (autoantibodies)	Prostatic secretory granules and vesicles composed of a lipid bilayer membrane and composite protein content	Consist of proteins that act in numerous enzymatic reactions, transport, structure, GTP activity, molecular chaperoning, and signal transduction	Diagnosis
ZAG	Glycoprotein	Induces lipid decline in adipocytes and therefore is implicated as possibly acting in cachexia	Diagnosis
CGRP	Neuropeptide	Vasodilatation and possibly regulation of protease secretion	Prognosis
PSP94	Nonglycosylated secretory peptide	In all probability acts as a growth and calcium regulator, apoptosis inducer, and an inhibitor of FSH	Diagnosis
Other methylated genes including RASSF1α, APC, RARB2, and CDH1	Hypermethylated DNA encoding for various peptides	Hypermethylation predictably inactivates gene transcription	Diagnosis

From: *J Cancer* (2010) 1:150–177. doi:10.7150/jca.1.150

Table 1.46 Relative risk (RR) related to family history of prostate cancer

Risk group	RR for prostate cancer (95 % CI)
Brother(s) with prostate cancer diagnosed at any age	3.14 (2.37–4.15)
Father with prostate cancer diagnosed at any age	2.35 (2.02–2.72)
One affected FDR diagnosed at any age	2.48 (2.25–2.74)
Affected FDRs diagnosed <65 years	2.87 (2.21–3.74)
Affected FDRs diagnosed ≥65 years	1.92 (1.49–2.47)
Second-degree relatives diagnosed at any age	2.52 (0.99–6.46)
Two or more affected FDRs diagnosed at any age	4.39 (2.61–7.39)

From: The National Cancer Institute (Adapted from Kiciński et al.)
CI confidence interval, *FDR* first-degree relative

Family History

- There is a twofold risk increase for developing prostate cancer when the father has it.
- There is a threefold risk increase for developing prostate cancer when one brother has it.
- Family history of breast cancer increases the risk of developing prostate cancer.
- Please see Table 1.46 for relative risk related to family history of prostate cancer.

Comorbidities

- Overweight people have an increased risk of developing prostate cancer.
- Men with high blood pressure are more likely to develop prostate cancer.
- Prostatitis may increase the risk of developing prostate cancer.
- Prostatic intraepithelial neoplasia (PIN) may be associated with increased risk of developing prostate cancer.

Age/Gender/Ethnicity/Nutrition/Lifestyle

- Prostate cancer is rare before age 40 and more frequent after age 50.
- 2 out of 3 prostate cancers occur after age 65.
- Prostate cancer is 60 % more frequent in African Americans.
- Poor screening increases the risk of developing prostate cancer.
- Men who have been around Agent Orange are at increased risk for developing prostate cancer.
- Men who drink too much alcohol are at increased risk for developing prostate cancer.
- Farmers are at increased risk for developing prostate cancer.
- Tire plant workers are at increased risk for developing prostate cancer.
- Painters are at increased risk for developing prostate cancer.
- Men who have been around cadmium are at increased risk for developing prostate cancer.

- Men who eat a diet high in fat, especially animal fat, are at increased risk for developing prostate cancer.
- Prostate cancer is most common in North America, northwestern Europe, Australia, and on the Caribbean islands. It is less common in Asia, Africa, and Central and South America.
- Some studies have found that high levels of physical activity, particularly in older men, may lower the risk for prostate cancer.
- There is concern that taking beta-carotene supplements may increase the risk of developing advanced prostate cancer.

Similarly:

- A recent study linked smoking to a small increase in the risk of death from prostate cancer.

Recommendations

- Eliminate/avoid/attenuate risk factors, if possible (please see above and below).
- Most major US medical organizations recommend that clinicians discuss the potential benefits and known harms of PSA screening with their patients, consider their patients' preferences, and individualize screening decisions. They generally agree that the most appropriate candidates for screening include men age 50 years or older who have a life expectancy of at least 10 years. These organizations include the American Academy of Family Physicians, American College of Physicians, American College of Preventive Medicine, and American Medical Association.
- The American Cancer Society and American Urological Association recommend offering PSA measurement and digital rectal examination to men annually beginning at age 50 years.
- The PSA test is more sensitive than the digital rectal examination for detecting prostate cancer. However, they complement each other.
- Variations of PSA screening, including the use of age-adjusted PSA cut points, free PSA, PSA density, PSA velocity, PSA slope, and PSA doubling time, have been proposed to improve detection of "clinically important" prostate cancer cases. However, no evidence suggests that any of these testing strategies improves health outcomes.
- PSA test results show the level of PSA detected in the blood. These results are usually reported as nanograms of PSA per milliliter (ng/mL) of blood. In the past, most doctors considered a PSA level below 4.0 ng/mL as normal. In one large study, however, prostate cancer was diagnosed in 15.2 % of men with a PSA level at or below 4.0 ng/mL. Fifteen percent of these men, or approximately 2.3 % overall, had high-grade cancers. In another study, 25 to 35 % of men who had a PSA level between 4.1 and 9.9 ng/mL and who underwent a prostate biopsy were found to have prostate cancer, meaning that 65 to 75 % of the remaining men did not have prostate cancer.
- Because PSA levels tend to increase with age, the use of age-specific PSA reference ranges has been suggested as a way of increasing the accuracy of PSA tests. However, age-specific reference ranges have not been generally favored because their use may lead to missing or delaying the detection of prostate cancer in as

many as 20 % of men in their 60s and 60 % of men in their 70s. Another compli-
cating factor is that studies to establish the normal range of PSA values have
been conducted primarily in white men. Expert opinions vary and there is no
clear consensus on the optimal PSA threshold for recommending a prostate
biopsy for men of any racial or ethnic group.

- There is no specific normal or abnormal PSA level. In addition, various factors,
  such as inflammation (e.g., prostatitis), can cause a man's PSA level to fluctuate.
  It is also common for PSA values to vary somewhat from laboratory to laboratory. Consequently, one abnormal PSA test result does not necessarily indicate
  the need for a prostate biopsy. In general, however, the higher a man's PSA level,
  the more likely it is that cancer is present. Furthermore, if a man's PSA level
  continues to rise over time, other tests may be needed.
- Consider the following table:

Age	<50		50–59		60–69		>70		
	Cancer	No cancer	Cancer	No cancer	Cancer	No cancer	Cancer	No cancer	
5th percentile	0.4	0.3	1.2	0.3	1.7	0.3	2.3	0.4	(ng/mL)
95th percentile	163.0	2.5	372.5	4.7	253.2	8.3	613.2	17.8	

1.23.1.2   Preventive Advice

Chemical

- 5-alpha reductase inhibitors including finasteride and dutasteride may reduce the
  overall risk of developing prostate cancer. If the patient is 55 or older, he does not have
  prostate cancer, and his PSA score is 3.0 or lower, the pros and cons of taking these
  drugs to prevent prostate cancer should be discussed. The Food and Drug Administration
  has warned that in some men these medications may actually increase the risk of getting
  a more serious form of prostate cancer (high-grade prostate cancer).
- Vitamin C may reduce the risk of developing prostate cancer.
- Vitamin E may reduce the risk of developing prostate cancer.
- Selenium may reduce the risk of developing prostate cancer.

Lifestyle

- Be informed about prostate cancer (please see Sect. 2.11).
- Maintain a healthy weight. Calculate BMI and, if needed, lose weight by increasing calorie output through exercising (please see Sect. 2.1) and decreasing calorie input by dieting.
- Do not smoke/stop smoking or chewing tobacco (please see Sect. 2.3).

- Control blood pressure.
- Get screened (please see above).

Nutrition

- Avoid:
  - Red meat
  - Delicatessen
  - Milk and dairy products in excess (particularly for African Americans)
  - Beta-carotene supplements

- Eat fruits and vegetables so that healthy levels of vitamins are maintained.
- Eat tomatoes, they contain lycodene which prevents prostate cancer.
- Adopt a diet that is:
  - High in omega-3 fatty acids
  - Low in fat
  - Similar to the traditional Japanese diet
  - Vegetarian

- Drink alcohol with moderation (please see Sect. 2.4).

1.24 Psoriasis

1.24.1 Risk Assessment and Prevention of Psoriasis

1.24.1.1 Risk Assessment

Genetic Markers

- Markers for psoriasis have been identified on at least 11 chromosomes (1, 3, 4, 6, 8, 10, 16, 17, 18, 19, and 20).
- On chromosome 6 the locus termed psoriasis susceptibility 1 (PSORS1) is considered the most important susceptibility locus. On the basis of association studies of three tightly linked susceptibility alleles, PSORS1 appears to be associated with up to 50 % of cases of psoriasis.
- The value of relative risk for psoriasis for HLA-B13 and HLA-B17 antigens is estimated at 5.3 and 7.7, respectively.
- HLA-Cw6 is a risk factor for psoriasis.
- Two genes activated by TNF-alpha—TNFAIP3 and TNIP1—show strong association with psoriasis.
- IL-12B, IL-23A, IL-23R, and IL-4/IL-13 are associated with psoriasis.
- Please see Table 1.47 for replicated genetic risk factors for psoriasis.

Table 1.47 Replicated genetic risk factors for psoriasis

Putative biological pathway	Gene or locus	Description	Locus	Expression in	(Putative) Function
Adaptive immunity	IL-23R	IL-23 receptor subunit	1p31.3	Macrophages, IL-23-activated dendritic cells (DCs), Th17 cells	Maturation T cells
Adaptive immunity	ERAP1	Endoplasmic reticulum aminopeptidase 1	5q15	Generally expressed	Several proposed functions, including trimming of peptide antigens for binding to major histocompatibility complex I
Adaptive immunity	IL-12B	IL-12/IL-23, subunit p40	5q31.1–q33.1	Th1, Th0, NK, monocyte, DC, and B-cell lines, induced in psoriasis-involved skin	Maturation T cells
Adaptive immunity	TNF	Tumor necrosis factor-α	6p21	Immune cells	Major proinflammatory cytokine involved in psoriasis
Adaptive immunity	TRAF3IP2	TRAF3-interacting protein 2	6q21	Generally expressed, induced in psoriasis-involved skin	Signaling adaptor involved in regulation of adaptive immunity
Adaptive immunity	IL-4, IL-13	IL-4, IL-13	5q31.1	Th2 cells	Modulate humoral immune response mediated by Th2 cells
Adaptive immunity	IL-23A/STAT2	IL-23, subunit p19	12q13.2	DCs and monocytes, induced in psoriasis-involved skin	Regulation T-cell activation
Adaptive immunity	IL-23A	IL-23, α-subunit p19	12q13.3	DCs and phagocytic cells	Involved in Th17 axis
Adaptive immunity	ZNF313/RNF114	Ring-finger protein 114	20q13.14	Generally expressed, strongest in skin, T lymphocytes, and DCs	Ubiquitination, regulation of immune responses
Adaptive immunity	HLA-C	MHC gene	6p21.33	All nucleated cells	Presenting antigens to immune cells

Barrier function skin	LCE3B and LCE3C	Late cornified envelope 3B and 3C	1q21.3	Epithelia and lesional PS skin	Barrier function skin
Barrier function skin	CDSN	Corneodesmosin	6p21	Epidermis, upregulated in psoriasis	Component of the cornified envelope
Barrier function skin	DEFB cluster	β-Defensins	8p23.1	Epithelium and male reproductive system	Antimicrobial and chemotactic functions
Barrier function skin	GJB2	Gap junction protein β2, connexin 26	13q11–q12	Skin, highly upregulated in psoriasis	Involved in gap junction formation
Innate immunity	IFIH1	IFN induced with helicase C domain 1, MDA5	2q24	Generally expressed, induced in psoriasis-involved skin	Rig-like helicase, involved in recognition RNA viruses
Innate immunity	REL	v-rel reticuloendotheliosis viral oncogene homologue	2p13	Blood, intestine, larynx, lymph node, thyroid, trachea	Transcription factor, member of the REL/NF-κB family
Innate immunity	TNIP1	TNAIP3-interacting protein 1	5q32–q33.1	Ubiquitously, stronger in blood lymphocytes, spleen, and skeletal muscle, induced in psoriasis-involved skin	Regulation of NF-κB signaling
Innate immunity	TNFAIP3	Tumor necrosis factor-α-induced protein 3/A20	6q23.3	Epithelia and lymphoid tissues	TNF-α inducible zinc finger protein that temporarily limits immune response by inhibiting NF-κB signaling
Innate immunity	IL-28RA	IL-29 receptor subunit	1p36.11	Lymph, lymph node	Receptor for IL-28A, IL-28B, and IL-29
Innate immunity	NFKBIA	NF of kappa light polypeptide gene enhancer in B-cell inhibitor; alpha	14q13.2	Generally expressed	Inhibiting NF-κB signaling
Innate immunity	FBXL19	F-box and leucine-rich repeat protein 19	16p11.2	Epithelia, brain, eye, lymph, bone, induced in psoriasis-involved skin	Putative inhibitor of demethylase activity to activate NF-κB

(continued)

Table 1.47 (continued)

Putative biological pathway	Gene or locus	Description	Locus	Expression in	(Putative) Function
Innate immunity	NOS2	Nitric oxide synthase 2, inducible	17q11.1	Immune system, cardiovascular system	Cytokine-inducible enzymes that catalyze the production of nitric oxide for immune defense against pathogens
Innate immunity	TYK2	Tyrosine kinase 2	19p13.2	Generally expressed	Tyrosine kinase, associates with cytoplasmic domains of type I and type II cytokine receptors
Not determined	SLC12A8	Solute carrier family 12, member 8	3q21	Generally expressed	Cation/chloride cotransporter, putatively involved in keratinocyte differentiation
Not determined	PTTG1	Pituitary tumor transforming gene	5q35.1	Generally expressed, not in skin and tissues from gastrointestinal tract	Multiple functions, roles in control of mitosis, cell transformation, DNA repair, and gene regulation
Not determined	CSMD1	CUB and Sushi multiple domains 1	8p23.2	Areas of regenerative growth, such as skin and epithelial cells	Tumor-repressor gene
Not determined	ADAM33	A disintegrin and metalloproteases metallopeptidase domain 33	20p13	Mesenchymal cells	Metalloprotease, linked to angiogenesis and remodeling
Not determined	SERPINB8	Serpin peptidase inhibitor clade B member 8	18q21.3	Skin, vascular tissue, connective tissue, upregulated in psoriasis	Serine proteinase inhibitor, regulates wide range of functions
Not determined	ZNF816A	Zinc finger protein 816A	19q13.41	Generally expressed	Regulatory function, belongs to the same family as ZNF313

From: *J Invest Dermatol* (2012) 132:2320–2331. doi:10.1038/jid.2012.167; published online 24 May 2012

Biochemical and Serological Markers

- T cells and TNF-alpha are involved in the pathogenesis of psoriasis.
- The biochemical basis for the pathogenesis of psoriasis can be attributed to both overexpression and underexpression of certain proteins in psoriatic lesions. The anomalies in protein expression can be classified as abnormal keratinocyte differentiation, keratinocyte hyperproliferation, and inflammation.
- Oxidative stress and increased free radical generation have been linked to skin inflammation in psoriasis.

Past Medical History

- Children and young adults with recurring infections, particularly strep throat, may be at increased risk for developing psoriasis.

Family History

- Psoriasis is passed down through families. About 40 % of people with psoriasis have a family member with the disease, although this may be an underestimate.
- A child with two affected parents has a 50 % chance of developing psoriasis. Siblings have a three- to sixfold risk.
- A child with one affected parent has a 10 % chance of developing psoriasis.

Comorbidities

- Inflammatory bowel diseases, such as ulcerative colitis and Crohn's disease, increase the risk of psoriasis by five to ten times.
- Seborrheic dermatitis is associated with psoriasis.
- Autoimmune disorders such as thyroiditis, rheumatoid arthritis, and lupus are associated with psoriasis.
- People with HIV/AIDS are more likely to develop psoriasis.
- Reiter's syndrome, sacroiliitis, and ankylosing spondylitis all seem to share common causes with psoriasis.
- Certain blistering diseases like bullous pemphigoid or pemphigus are weakly associated with psoriasis.
- People undergoing cancer chemotherapy are at increased risk for developing psoriasis.
- Some medicines, including antimalarial drugs, beta-blockers, and lithium, can trigger psoriasis.

Similarly:

- Up to 1/3 of people with psoriasis may also have psoriatic arthritis.
- Severe psoriasis doubles the risk of kidney diseases.

Age/Gender/Ethnicity/Nutrition/Lifestyle

- Psoriasis most commonly begins between ages 15 and 35.
- The sex incidence of psoriasis is equal.
- In the United States, the prevalence among blacks (0.45– 0.7 %) is far lower than that in the remainder of the US population (1.4–4.6 %).
- The prevalence of psoriasis in central Europe is 0 %, in the Samoan population approximately 1.5 % and 12 % in Arctic Kasach'ye.
- Smoking tobacco increases the risk of developing psoriasis and may increase the severity of the disease.
- High stress levels may increase the risk of developing psoriasis.
- Excess weight increases the risk of inverse psoriasis (lesions appear in intertriginous areas, where scaling is minimal).

Recommendations

- Eliminate/avoid/attenuate risk factors, if possible (please see above and below).

1.24.1.2 Preventive Advice

Chemical

- Avoid certain medications such as antimalarial drugs, beta-blockers, and lithium.
- Omega-3 fatty acids found in fish oil supplements may help in preventing psoriasis (up to 3 g/day).
- Vitamin B1 may decrease the risk of developing psoriasis.
- Vitamin B12 may decrease the risk of developing psoriasis.
- Vitamin C may decrease the risk of developing psoriasis.
- Folic acid may decrease the risk of developing psoriasis.

Lifestyle

- Exercise (please see Sect. 2.1).
- Avoid stress (please see Sect. 2.2) and anxiety.
- Do not smoke/stop smoking or chewing tobacco (please see Sect. 2.3).
- Maintain a healthy weight. Lose weight, if necessary, by increasing calorie output through exercising and decreasing calorie input through dieting.
- Avoid skin infections and injuries.
- Avoid intense sun exposure.
- Keep skin moist.
- Avoid skin injuries (picking, cuts, or scrapes).
- Avoid infection.

Nutrition

• Eat a healthy diet including a variety fruits and vegetables of all colors, whole grains, and nuts.

1.25   Restless Legs Syndrome

1.25.1   *Risk Assessment and Prevention of Restless Leg Syndrome (RLS)*

1.25.1.1   Risk Assessment

Genetic Markers

• Loci on the following chromosomes are associated with RLS: 2p, 9p, 12q, 14q, 15q, 20p, and 16p12.1.
• The following genes MEIS1, BTBD9, MAP2K5, and PTPRD are associated with RLS.
• There are significant associations between RLS and intronic variants in the homeobox gene MEIS1, the BTBD9 gene encoding a BTB(POZ) domain, as well as variants in a third locus containing the genes encoding mitogen-activated protein kinase MAP2K5 and the transcription factor LBXCOR1 on chromosomes 2p, 6p, and 15q, respectively. Each genetic variant is associated with more than 50 % increase in risk for RLS, with the combined allelic variants conferring more than half of the risk.
• Please see Table 1.48 for genes associated with RLS susceptibility and their possible roles.

Biochemical and Serological Markers

• Please see Table 1.49 for the laboratory profile of RLS.

Past Medical History

• The use of certain medications such as calcium channel blockers, lithium, or neuroleptics increases the risk of developing RLS.
• Withdrawal from sedatives increases the risk of developing RLS.
• The use of some recreational drugs such as ecstasy increases the risk of developing RLS.
• Discontinuing benzodiazepines increases the risk of developing RLS.
• Opioid detoxification has been associated with the development of RLS.

Table 1.48 Genes associated with RLS susceptibility and their possible roles

Gene	Development	Neurobiology	Others	Possible associated symptoms
MEIS1 (homeodomain transcription factor)	Proximodistal limb axis development, neuronal differentiation, and hindbrain patterning	Expressed strongly in the substantia nigra and red nucleus; could work with iron within these structures known to regulate motor control	Peripheral expression (including skeletal muscles)	Urge to move and/or periodic limb movements during sleep
BTBD9 (zinc finger transcription factor)	Role unknown, but family implicated in a multitude of developmental events, including gastrulation, cell fate, and limb formation	Widespread brain expression	Notable liver expression; affects ferritin level, iron storage	Primary effects on periodic limb movements during sleep in individuals with RLS
MAP2K5 (kinase)	Interacts/activates MAPK7/ERK5; involved in growth factor-stimulated cell proliferation and muscle cell differentiation	Widespread brain expression	Widespread peripheral expression (including the skeletal muscle and liver)	Unknown
LBXCOR1 (homeodomain transcription factor)	Discrete developmental expression at the midbrain–hindbrain border and in the spinal cord; with Lbx1, regulates the GABAergic phenotype of dorsal horn interneurons	Selective brain/spinal cord expression	None	Sensory and pain perception; discomfort or pain in the legs

From: *Nat Genet* (2007) 39: 938–939, doi:10.1038/ng0807-938

Table 1.49 Laboratory profile of RLS

	RLS ($n=59$)	Non-RLS ($n=655$)	Significance[a]
Hemoglobin (g/dL^{-1})	13.7±1.2	13.9±1.4	0.3
Iron (µg/dL^{-1})	105.7±37.8	102.7±36.0	0.55
Ferritin (ng/mL^{-1})	119.4±106.0	114.6±121.1	0.77
Ferritin (<50/ng/mL^{-1}, %)	18.6	22.1	0.36
Transferrin (mg/dL^{-1})	236.7±39.9	238.2±44.1	0.8
TIBC (µg/dL^{-1})	326.6±51.0	332.0±52.3	0.45
BUN (mg/dL^{-1})	15.4±4.6	16.0±5.3	0.44
Creatinine (mg/dL^{-1})	1.1±0.2	1.1±0.3	0.58
Renal insufficiency (%)[b]	49.1	43.5	0.41
Glucose (mg/dL^{-1})	106.9±18.7	110.0±27.3	0.38
HbA1C (%)	6.0±0.6	6.0±0.9	0.71
Diabetes mellitus (%)[c]	15.3	15.4	0.98
Total cholesterol (mg/dL^{-1})	210.7±36.1	204.7±37.8	0.25
T3R (ng/L^{-1})	133.6±16.4	130.2±19.0	0.19
Free T4 (ng/dL^{-1})	9.0±1.6	9.0±1.9	0.85
TSH (µIU/dL^{-1})	3.4±2.5	3.1±3.4	0.55
Vitamin B$_{12}$ (pg/dL^{-1})	674.0±311.2	655.1±352.0	0.69
Folate (ng/dL^{-1})	13.1±17.5	12.3±11.8	0.64
CRP (mg/dL^{-1})	0.19±0.36	0.23±0.65	0.61

From: *J Sleep Res* 19:87–92. doi:10.1111/j.1365-2869.2009.00739.x

TIBC total iron-binding capacity, *CRP* C-reactive protein, *BUN* blood urea nitrogen, *HbA1C* hemoglobin A1C, *TSH* thyroid-stimulating hormone

[a]Age- and gender-adjusted ANOVA for continuous variables or Pearson's chi-squared test for dichotomous variables

[b]Ccr $\leq$59 mL/min^{-1} 1.73 m^2

[c]Fasting glucose $\geq$126 mg/dL^{-1}

Family History

- RLS is commonly passed down in families. More than 60 % of cases of RLS are familial.
- Having one child nearly doubles the risk of having RLS, two children triples the risk, and three or more children increases the odds ratio to 3.57.

Comorbidities

- Chronic kidney disease increases the risk of developing RLS.
- Diabetes increases the risk of developing RLS.
- Parkinson's disease increases the risk of developing RLS.
- Peripheral neuropathy increases the risk of developing RLS.
- Antidopaminergic antiemetics increase the risk of developing RLS.

- Certain antihistamines increase the risk of developing RLS.
- Serotonin antidepressants increase the risk of developing RLS.
- Antipsychotics and certain anticonvulsants increase the risk of developing RLS.
- H2 histamine blockers increase the risk of developing RLS.

Age/Gender/Ethnicity/Nutrition/Lifestyle

- The risk of developing RLS increases with age.
- RLS is more common in women than men.
- Sleep deprivation increases the risk of developing RLS.
- Iron deficiency increases the risk of developing RLS.
- Coffee, alcohol, and tobacco can trigger RLS.
- Pregnancy increases the risk of developing RLS, particularly in the last trimester.

Recommendations

- Eliminate/avoid/attenuate risk factors, if possible (please see above and below).
- Treat the underlying condition when there is one.

1.25.1.2 Preventive Advice

Chemical

- Avoid recreational drugs or medicines which have triggered the first episode of RLS.
- Vitamin B12 may decrease the risk of developing RLS.
- Vitamin E may decrease the risk of developing RLS.
- Folic acid may decrease the risk of developing RLS.
- Magnesium may decrease the risk of developing RLS.
- Calcium may decrease the risk of developing RLS.
- Iron may decrease the risk of developing RLS.

Lifestyle

- Get regular exercise (please see Sect. 2.1).
- Reduce stress (please see Sect. 2.2).
- Do not smoke/quit smoking or chewing tobacco (please see Sect. 2.3).
- Sleep better by sticking to a regular sleep schedule or engaging in sleeping health promotion programs (please see Sect. 2.2).

Nutrition

- If at risk, avoid or cut back on caffeine.
- If at risk, avoid alcohol.

1.26 Rheumatoid Arthritis

1.26.1 Risk Assessment and Prevention of Rheumatoid Arthritis (RA)

1.26.1.1 Risk Assessment

Genetic Markers

- HLA-DR4 is associated with RA. People with this genetic marker have a fivefold greater chance of developing RA than people without the marker.
- Two alleles, DRB1*0401 and DRB1*0404, primarily account for the DR4 association with RA in Caucasians.
- A DR1 allele is present in many of Caucasian RA patients who are negative for DR4 alleles.
- 80 % of whites with RA express the HLA-DR1 or HLA-DR4 subtypes,
- Other genes that have a connection to RA are STAT4, TRAF1 and C5, and PTPN22.
- Other regions of the major histocompatibility complex may confer susceptibility to more severe disease by causing a specific arthrogenic peptide to be presented to CD4+ T cells.
- As of 2012, approximately 16 % of phenotypic variance has been accounted for genetically. Please see graph below:

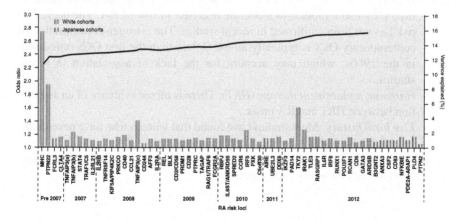

RA genetic susceptibility loci and cumulative proportion of observed variance in disease susceptibility (From: *Nat Rev Rheumatol* (2013);9:141–153. doi:10.1038/nrrheum.2012.237)

Biochemical and Serological Markers

- Autoantibodies to IgGFc, known as rheumatoid factor (RF), and antibodies to citrullinated peptides (ACPA) are associated with RA.
- The most common tests for ACPAs are the anti-CCP (cyclic citrullinated peptide) test and the anti-MCV assay (antibodies against mutated citrullinated vimentin).
- A serological point-of-care test (POCT) for the early detection of RA has been developed. This assay combines the detection of rheumatoid factor and anti-MCV for the diagnosis of rheumatoid arthritis and shows a sensitivity of 72 % and specificity of 99.7 %.
- Regardless of the exact trigger of RA, the result is an immune system that is geared up to promote inflammation in the joints and occasionally other tissues of the body. Lymphocytes are activated, and chemical messengers (cytokines, such as tumor necrosis factor/TNF, interleukin-1/IL-1, and interleukin-6/IL-6) are expressed in the inflamed areas.
- Presence of leukopenia increases the risk of developing RA.
- Elevated ESR (erythrocyte sedimentation rate) increases the risk of developing RA.
- Many biomarkers have been studied for the diagnosis of RA. Please see Table 1.50.

Past Medical History

- Approximately 10–20 % of patients with early RA have serologic evidence of recent infective agents as triggers of RA, but there is not one single putative microbial trigger.
- Hormone changes and events in women's life are associated with RA as follows:

  – *Oral contraceptives (OC)*: Early studies found that women who had ever used OCs had a modest to moderate decrease in risk of RA. The decreased risk has not been confirmed in recent studies. The estrogen concentration of contemporary OCs is typically 80–90 % less than the first OCs introduced in the 1960s, which may account for the lack of association in recent studies.
  – *Hormone replacement therapy (HRT)*: There is mixed evidence of an association between HRT and RA onset.
  – *Live birth history*: Most studies have found that women who have never had a live birth have a slight to moderately increased risk of RA.
  – *Breastfeeding*: Recent population-based studies have found that RA is less common among women who breastfeed.

– *Menstrual history*: At least two studies have observed that women with irregular menses or a truncated menstrual history (e.g., early menopause) have an increased risk of RA. Because women with polycystic ovarian syndrome (PCOS) have an increased risk of RA, the association with an aberrant menstrual history may result from PCOS.

Table 1.50 Biomarkers in rheumatoid arthritis vs. other diseases

Biomarker in RA	Other diseases
Autoantibodies	
RF	Sjogren's syndrome, crioglobulinemia, SLE
AKA, AFA, APF	ReA
Anti-CCP	AS, ReA, PsA, SLE, CREST, systemic sclerosis, Sjogren's syndrome
MCV	OA, UA, PsA, SLE, Sjogren's syndrome, scleroderma, AS, systemic sclerosis, viral hepatitis B, tuberculosis, PMR
Inflammatory markers	
Cytokines\inhibitors (e.g., TNF-α, IL-1, IL-6, IL-8, IL-16)	OA, GOUT, PMR, ReA, acute crystal arthritis
Calprotectin	OA
E-selectin	OA
sVCAM, ICAM	OA, IA, SLE
Thioredoxin	OA, GOUT, ReA
Synovium/cartilage markers	
Hyaluronic acid	OA
COMP	JCA, OA, SLE, ReA, PsA, Scleroderma, vasculitis, Sjogren's syndrome, Raynaud's syndrome
Aggrecan/CS846-epitope	OA
Glc-Gal-PYD	Paget's disease
MMPs	IA, OA, SLE
C2C, C1,2C	AO, PsA
Bone markers	
BSP	PsA
Immunological markers	
Regulatory T cells	PsA, JIA, spondyloarthropathies, ReA

From: *Rheumatol Rep* (2010) 2:e3. doi:10.4081/rr.2010.e3

RF rheumatoid factor, *AKA* antikeratin antibodies, *AFA* antifilaggrin antibodies, *APF* antiperinuclear factor, *MCV* antimutated citrullinated vimentin, *COMP* cartilage oligomeric protein, *Glc-Gal-PYD* urinary glucosyl-galactosyl-pyridinoline, *MMPs* matrix metalloproteases, *BSP* bone sialoprotein, *SLE* systemic lupus erythematosus, *ReA* reactive arthritis, *AS* ankylosing spondylitis, *PsA* psoriatic arthritis, *OA* osteoarthritis, *UA* undifferentiated arthritis, *PMR* polymyalgia rheumatica, *IA* inflammatory arthritis, *JCA* juvenile chronic arthritis, *JIA* juvenile idiopathic arthritis

Family History

- A positive family history for RA increases the risk of developing RA.
- In monozygotic twins, there is a more than 30 % concordance rate for RA.

Comorbidities

- Diabetes mellitus increases the risk of developing RA.
- Chronic lung disease increases the risk of developing RA.
- There are positive associations between RA and non-Hodgkin's lymphoma, Hodgkin's disease, and lung cancer.
- There is a positive association between RA and Graves' disease.
- Raynaud's phenomenon can be associated with RA.

Similarly:

- People with RA are at higher risk for developing cardiovascular disease (such as angina, heart attack, and stroke).
- People with RA are at higher risk for developing anemia.
- People with RA are at higher risk for developing infections (particularly in joints).
- People with RA are at higher risk for developing osteoporosis.
- An increased incidence of lymphoproliferative malignancies (such as leukemia and multiple myeloma) has been reported among people with RA.
- People with RA have a slightly elevated risk of developing melanoma.

Age/Gender/Ethnicity/Nutrition/Lifestyle

- Rheumatoid arthritis can occur at any age but starts usually after 40.
- Women are three times more likely to develop RA than men.
- In women, rheumatoid arthritis usually begins between the ages of 30 and 60.
- Smoking cigarettes increases the risk of developing RA.
- Emotional and physical trauma and stress (e.g., from an infection) may contribute to developing RA.
- Silicate exposure increases the risk of developing RA.
- Alcoholism increases the risk of developing RA.

Recommendations

- Eliminate/avoid/attenuate risk factors, if possible (please see above and below).

1.26.1.2 Preventive Advice

Chemical

- Fish oil may help in decreasing the risk of developing RA (please note that it can interfere with medications).
- Vitamins B6, B9, and B12 may help in decreasing the risk of developing RA.
- Vitamin C may help in decreasing the risk of developing RA.
- Vitamin D may help in decreasing the risk of developing RA.
- Vitamin E may help in decreasing the risk of developing RA.
- Calcium may help in decreasing the risk of developing RA.

Lifestyle

- Get regular exercise (please see Sect. 2.1).
- Practice tai chi.
- Reduce stress (please see Sect. 2.2).
- Do not smoke/quit smoking or chewing tobacco (please see Sect. 2.3).
- Control blood sugar.
- Stay lean. Calculate BMI and lose weight by exercising and dieting, if necessary.
- Breastfeed babies.

Nutrition

- Drink alcohol with moderation (please see Sect. 2.4).
- Eat a healthy diet particularly including plant oils.

1.27 Sarcoidosis

1.27.1 Risk Assessment and Prevention of Sarcoidosis

1.27.1.1 Risk Assessment

Genetic Markers

- The HLA (human leukocyte antigen) system is associated with sarcoidosis as follows (Table 1.51):

Table 1.51 Summary of HLA association studies of sarcoidosis

HLA	Risk alleles	Finding
HLA-A	A*1	Susceptibility
HLA-B	B*8	Susceptibility in several populations
HLA-DPB1	*0201	Not associated with sarcoidosis
HLA-DQB1	*0201	Protection, Löfgren's syndrome, mild disease in several populations
	*0602	Susceptibility/disease progression in several groups
HLA-DRB1	*0301	Acute onset/good prognosis in several groups
	*04	Protection in several populations
	*1101	Susceptibility in whites and African Americans. Stage II/III chest X-ray
HLA-DRB3	*1501	Associated with Löfgren's syndrome
	*0101	Susceptibility/disease progression in whites

From: *Proc Am Thorac Soc* (2007) 4(1):108–166

- Other markers include:

    - Angiotensin-converting enzyme 17q23: increased risk for ID and DD genotypes 23, 24, 132–134 and/or moderate association between II genotype and radiographic progression
    - Clara cell 10 kD protein 11q 12–13 C: allele: associated with sarcoidosis and with progressive disease at 3-year follow-up
    - Complement receptor 1 1q32. GG genotype for the Pro1827Arg(C-5,507-G) polymorphism: significantly associated with sarcoidosis
    - Cystic fibrosis transmembrane regulator 7q31.2: R75Q: increased risk for sarcoidosis
    - HSPA1L heat shock protein 70 1 like (alias heat 6p21.3. HSP-2437 cm^3): associated with susceptibility to sarcoidosis
    - IL-1 2q14: the IL-1 889 1.1 genotype: increased risk for sarcoidosis
    - IL-18 11q22: genotype 607CA: increased risk for sarcoidosis
    - IFN-9p22: IFNA17 polymorphism (551 T→G) and IFNA10[60A] IFN-17 [551G] haplotype: increased risk for sarcoidosis
    - Toll-like receptor 4 9q32 B Asp299Gly and Thre399Ile mutations: associated with chronic disease
    - TGF 19q13.2: TGF-2 59941 allele, TGF-3 4875 A, and 17369 C alleles: associated with chest X-ray detection of fibrosis
    - TNF-6p21.3: genotype 857T allele: associated with sarcoidosis
    - Vitamin D receptor 12q12–14 BsmI allele: elevated in sarcoidosis patients

Biochemical and Serological Markers

- Please see Table 1.52 for the association of biomarkers with sarcoidosis.

Table 1.52 Association of biomarkers with sarcoidosis

Investigator	Patients controls	Biomarker/summary	ROC curve analysis cutoff values	Specificity/sensitivity diagnostic accuracy	Limitations
Ziegenhagen et al.	77 50	TNF-α release from alveolar macrophages and serum level of sIL-2R are prognostic markers for sarcoidosis patients	No	Not estimated	No serial measurements/no ROC curve analysis/cutoff values
Ziegenhagen et al.	73 48	BAL and serological parameters reflect the severity of sarcoidosis	No	Not estimated High predictive value for neopterin + sIL-2R	No serial measurement/no ROC curve analysis/cutoff values
Grutters et al.	47	Positive correlation between sIL-2R serum levels and the disease activity and severity in patients with sarcoidosis	No	Not estimated	Small number of patients with serial measurement/no ROC curve analysis/cutoff values
Rothkrantz-Kos et al.	144 282	Potential usefulness of inflammatory markers to monitor respiratory functional impairment in sarcoidosis	Yes sIL-2R: 750 U/mL sIL-2R: 1,300 U/mL	sIL-2R: 94–82 % sIL-2R: 82–94 %	Discrepancies between treated and untreated patients/no serial measurements/retrospective study/no correlation with radiological findings
Hashimoto et al.	26	Correlation of plasma MCP-1 and MIP-1a levels with disease activity and clinical course of sarcoidosis patients	No	Not estimated	Small number of patients/no ROC curve analysis/cutoff values/no determination of the cytokines' cellular sources
Iyonaga et al.	47 10	MIP-1 serum levels estimate the activity of granuloma formation in sarcoidosis	No	Not estimated	Small number of patients/no ROC curve analysis/cutoff values/no correlation with radiological findings
Kobayashi et al.	47	Serum KL-6 for the evaluation of active pneumonitis in pulmonary sarcoidosis	No	Not estimated	Small number of patients/no follow-up laboratory data

(continued)

Table 1.52 (continued)

Investigator	Patients controls	Biomarker/summary	ROC curve analysis cutoff values	Specificity/sensitivity diagnostic accuracy	Limitations
Hermans et al.	117 117	Serum CC16 levels, a marker of the integrity of the air–blood barrier in sarcoidosis	No	Not estimated	Non-ILD-specific marker/potential influence by tobacco smoking/ poor discriminative value
Janssen et al.	79 38	Elevated serum CC16, KL-6, and SP-D levels reflect pulmonary disease severity and prognosis in sarcoidosis patients	Yes CC16: 12.7 ng/ mL KL-6: 223 U/ mL SP-D: 91.7 ng/ mL	CC16: 84–73–73 % KL-6: 84–86–86 % SP-D: 84–66–66 %	Non-ILD-specific markers/ Retrospective study/No serial measurement

From: *Respir Res* (2005):6(1):78. Published online 2005 21 July. doi:10.1186/1465-9921-6-78

Abbreviations: *CC16* clara cell protein 16, *ILD* interstitial lung disease, *KL-6* Krebs von den Lungen-6, *MCP-1* monocyte chemoattractant protein-1, *MIP-1a* monocyte inflammatory protein-1a, *ROC* receiver operating characteristic, *sIL-2R* soluble interleukin-2 receptor, *SP* surfactant protein, *TNF-α* tumor necrosis factor-alpha

Family History

- A person with a close blood relative who has sarcoidosis is nearly five times as likely to develop the disease.

Comorbidities

- Infectious diseases: HCV infection is the infectious disease most commonly associated with sarcoidosis.
- Neoplastic disorders as follows:

  - Lung cancer and non-Hodgkin's lymphoma: the relative risk is doubled during the first decade of disease.
  - Melanoma: elevated risk of developing sarcoidosis.
  - Non-melanoma skin cancer: elevated risk of developing sarcoidosis.
  - Liver cancer: elevated risk of developing sarcoidosis.
  - Lymphomas: elevated risk of developing sarcoidosis.

- Immunologic-inflammatory diseases such as:

  - Lupus erythematosus: elevated risk of developing sarcoidosis.
  - Myasthenia gravis: elevated risk of developing sarcoidosis.
  - Primary biliary cirrhosis: elevated risk of developing sarcoidosis.

- In women, a substantial association between thyroid disease and sarcoidosis has been reported. The association is less marked but still significant for males.
- Sarcoidosis has been associated with celiac disease.

Age/Gender/Ethnicity/Nutrition/Lifestyle

- Sarcoidosis usually occurs between the ages of 20 and 40.
- Women are slightly more likely to develop sarcoidosis than men.
- African Americans have a higher incidence of sarcoidosis than Caucasians.
- Worldwide, sarcoidosis is more frequent in families of Asian, German, Irish, Puerto Rican, and Scandinavian origin.

Similarly:

- Sarcoidosis is likely to be more severe in blacks and to cause skin problems in this population.
- People with Japanese ancestry are more likely to develop eye or cardiac complications from the disease.

Recommendations

- Eliminate/avoid/attenuate risk factors, if possible (please see above and below).

1.27.1.2 Preventive Advice

Chemical

- The following supplements may help:
  - Supplements containing the antioxidant vitamins A, C, and E; the B-complex vitamins; and trace minerals such as magnesium, calcium, zinc, and selenium.
  - Omega-3 fatty acids.
  - Bromelain. Please note that it can increase the risk of bleeding and may interact with other medications.
  - Probiotic supplement (containing *Lactobacillus acidophilus*).

Lifestyle

General hygienic precautions may help:

- Get regular exercise (please see Sect. 2.1).
- Reduce stress (please see Sect. 2.2).
- Do not smoke/quit smoking or chewing tobacco (please see Sect. 2.3).

Nutrition

Improve overall nutritional intake:

- Eat antioxidant foods, including fruits (such as blueberries, cherries, and tomatoes) and vegetables (such as squash and bell peppers).
- Include foods rich in magnesium and low in calcium, such as barley, bran, corn, rye, oats, brown rice, avocado, banana, and potato.
- Avoid refined foods, such as white breads, pastas, and sugar.
- Eat fewer red meats and more lean meats, cold-water fish, tofu (soy, if no allergy), or beans for protein.
- Use healthy oils, such as olive oil or vegetable oil.
- Reduce or eliminate trans-fatty acids, found in commercially baked goods such as cookies, crackers, cakes, French fries, onion rings, donuts, processed foods, and margarine.
- Avoid caffeine and alcohol.
- Drink six to eight glasses of filtered water daily.

1.28 Stomach Cancer (Hereditary Diffuse Gastric Cancer)

1.28.1 Risk Assessment and Prevention of Hereditary Diffuse Gastric Cancer (HDGC)

1.28.1.1 Risk Assessment

Genetic Markers

- BRCA1 and BRCA2: Individuals who have inherited these genetic mutations are at an increased risk for stomach cancer.
- Mutations in the E-cadherin (CDH1) gene are a well-documented cause of HDGC.
- CDH1 mutations cause only 1–3 % of all gastric cancers, and in families with a strong history of diffuse gastric cancer, only 1/3–1/2 are due to CDH1 mutations.
- The CDH1 mutations include small insertions and deletions, splice site mutations, and three nonconservative amino acid substitutions (A298T, W409R, and R732Q).
- For people with the CDH1 mutation, the estimated cumulative risk of developing gastric cancer by age 80 years is 80 % for both men and women.
- Please see Table 1.53 for gastric cancer in hereditary cancer syndromes.

Table 1.53 Gastric cancer in hereditary cancer syndromes

Syndromes	Genes involved	Gastric cancer risk (%)	References
Hereditary diffuse gastric cancer syndrome (HDGC)	*CDH1*	67–83	Kaurah et al. Pharoah et al.
Hereditary nonpolyposis colorectal cancer (HNPCC)	*MLH1, MSH2, MSH6, PMS2*	2–30	Koornstra et al.
Peutz-Jeghers syndrome (PJS)	*STK11*	29	van Lier et al.
Hereditary breast/ovarian cancer syndrome (HBOC)	*BRCA1*	5.5	Thompson and Easton Brose et al.
	BRCA2	2.6	Breast Cancer Linkage Consortium Easton et al.
Familial adenomatous polyposis (FAP)	*APC*	2.1–4.2[a]	Park et al. Iwama et al.
Juvenile polyposis syndrome (JPS)[b]	*SMAD4, BMPR1A*	N/A	–
Li-Fraumeni syndrome (LFS)[b]	*TP53*	N/A	–

From: *Gen Med* (2011) 13:651–657. doi:10.1097/GIM.0b013e31821628b6
[a]This increased risk is for the Korean and Japanese populations. In other ethnicities, the risk is the same as the general population
[b]The estimate of the gastric cancer risk has not been calculated for these conditions

Biochemical and Serological Markers

- Currently available biomarkers used for prognosis and recurrence risk include:
  - CEA
  - CA 19.9
  - CA 72.4
  - Cytokeratins (CYFRA, 21.1, TPA, TPS)
  - Beta subunits of HCG

Past Medical History

- A polyp larger than 2 cm in the stomach increases the risk of developing HDGC.
- Vagotomy is a risk factor for stomach cancer.
- Partial gastrectomy is a risk factor for stomach cancer.

Family History

- In up to 10 % of hereditary nonpolyposis colon cancer (HNPCC) families gastric cancers can be found.
- A parent who carries a CDH1 mutation will have a 50 % chance of passing on the mutation to each of the children. Most CDH1 families will have several generations of relatives affected, but it is possible to have a carrier parent who has not been diagnosed with gastric cancer or breast cancer.
- People with familial adenomatous polyposis are at increased risk for developing HDGC.
- There is increased risk of developing HGSC if in the family there is:
  - At least two cases of stomach cancer, with at least one being diffuse gastric cancer and diagnosed before age 50
  - At least three cases of stomach cancer at any age, with at least one being diffuse gastric cancer
  - A person diagnosed with diffuse gastric cancer before age 45
  - A person diagnosed with both diffuse gastric cancer and lobular breast cancer
  - A person diagnosed with diffuse gastric cancer and another family member diagnosed with lobular breast cancer
  - A person diagnosed with diffuse gastric cancer and another family member diagnosed with signet cell adenocarcinoma of the colon

Comorbidities

- People with Li–Fraumeni syndrome are at increased risk for developing HDGC.
- People with Peutz–Jeghers syndrome are at increased risk for developing HDGC.
- Atrophic gastritis is a risk factor for stomach cancer.

Table 1.54 Cumulative risk of gastric and breast cancer in E-Cadherin/CDH1 mutation carriers

Age (years)	Male gastric cancer (%)	Female gastric cancer (%)	Female breast cancer (%)
30	4	4	0
40	9	21	3
50	21	46	10
60	43	64	19
70	52	71	29
80	67	83	39

Data adapted from: *ASCO Educational Sessions* (2002) pp. 116–125

- Menetrier's disease is a risk factor for stomach cancer.
- Stomach polyps are a risk factor for HDGC.
- Pernicious anemia is a risk factor for stomach cancer (it multiplies it two to three times).
- Infection with *Helicobacter pylori* increases the risk of developing HDGC.
- Chronic gastritis increases the risk of developing HDGC.
- Obesity has been linked to an increased risk of stomach cancer.

Similarly:

- People with HDGC are at higher risk for developing colorectal cancer.
- Women with HDGC are at high risk for developing lobular breast cancer.
- There is a cumulative risk of gastric and breast cancer: Please see Table 1.54.

Age/Gender/Ethnicity/Nutrition/Lifestyle

- The average age of onset of HDGC is 38 years.
- A diet high in salty and smoked foods increases the risk of developing HDGC.
- A diet low in fruits and vegetables increases the risk of developing HDGC.
- Eating foods contaminated with aflatoxin fungus increases the risk of developing HDGC.
- Smoking increases the risk of developing HDGC.
- Stomach cancer is more common in Japan, Korea, parts of Eastern Europe, and Latin America.
- Working in the coal, metal, or rubber industries is a risk factor for developing stomach cancer. Chemicals that are released in these environments have been linked to the development of the disease.

Recommendations

- Eliminate/avoid/attenuate risk factors, if possible (please see above and below).
- For those individuals carrying known CDH1 mutations, but without evidence for gastric cancer, recommendations include intensive and regular screening with endoscopy every 6–12 months with multiple biopsies of any suspicious site as well as random biopsies throughout the stomach.

- Individuals from HDGC families should also discuss the option of prophylactic total gastrectomy. The lifetime risk of stomach cancer is very high in CDH1 carriers, and without a proven effective screening test, surgery is a realistic and reasonable option. Gastrectomy in CDH1 gene carriers has to date been performed in only a very few patients. However, the Stanford experience suggests that this may be the best approach to prevention at the current time.
- HDGC patients seriously considering prophylactic gastrectomy should make sure their surgeon is well experienced in this procedure and is knowledgeable about HDGC cancer risks to ensure that the best technique is chosen while minimizing the risk of surgical complications.
- Women in families with HDGC and carrying mutations in the CDH1 gene have a significant risk to develop lobular breast cancer, with lifetime estimates from 20 to 40 %. The correct approach to screening for lobular breast cancer in women with HDGC is not known, but it is reasonable to adapt the screening recommendations for women at high genetic risk of breast cancer for other reasons such as carrying a BRCA1 or BRCA2 mutation.

1.28.1.2 Preventive Advice

Chemical

- People with chronic infection with *H. pylori* bacteria should be treated.
- Using aspirin (ASA), may lower the risk of stomach cancer and colon cancer. However, it can also cause serious internal bleeding and other problems. Most doctors think that the lower cancer risk is an added benefit for patients who take ASA for other problems such as arthritis, but they do not recommend taking it just to reduce the risk of cancer.
- Vitamin A may reduce the risk of developing HDGC.
- Vitamin C may reduce the risk of developing HDGC.
- Vitamin E may reduce the risk of developing HDGC.
- Selenium may reduce the risk of developing HDGC.

Lifestyle

- Know about gastric cancer (please see Sect. 2.13).
- Control weight: calculate BMI and if necessary lose weight by increasing caloric output through exercising (please see Sect. 2.1) and reducing caloric intake through dieting.
- Do not smoke/quit smoking or chewing tobacco (please see Sect. 2.3).

Nutrition

- Minimize the intake of salty and smoked foods.
- A diet high in fresh fruits and vegetables can lower stomach cancer risk. Citrus fruits (such as oranges, lemons, and grapefruits) may be helpful. The American Cancer Society recommends at least five servings of vegetables and fruits each day (please see Sect. 2.5), as well as whole-grain foods like breads, cereals, pasta, rice, and beans.
- Limit red meat intake.

Conclusions

The cornerstone of prevention is awareness, and health risk assessments are the gateway to health promotion programs aimed mostly at inducing long-lasting healthy behavior change. Patients and physicians of the entire US population should create custom-designed health pathways together.

From the examples included in this book, a process can be formulated regarding risk management of all diseases. It is as follows:

- Try and identify specific risks before symptoms appear. Taking a science-based and well-designed (including genetic tests, biochemical and serological markers) health risk assessment would be the first step.
- Adopt specific measures to address these risks (avoiding/eliminating/attenuating them).
- Follow the general guidelines of a healthy lifestyle, which includes:

  - Maintaining a normal weight
  - Exercising regularly
  - Never starting to smoke/stopping tobacco use
  - Sleeping well
  - Limiting stress/knowing how to handle it
  - Drinking alcohol with moderation (preferably red wine)
  - Eating wholesome food (the Mediterranean diet is the diet of choice)
  - Using nutritional supplements (vitamins and minerals) judiciously

Health pathways should include the health promotion guidelines outlined above as well as improving other important dimensions of life such as relationships (professional and personal—spouse/partner, family, friends, pets), economic situation, living environment, immunization, hygiene, habits, hobbies, etc. They should be reviewed alone or with professional help and adjusted on a yearly basis or more frequently, if needed, from birth to death.

I hope that this book will be a useful tool to medical professionals in their daily practice as well.

It is an embryo. If it triggers more research and work along the lines, it suggests my goal will have been reached and some ground broken. My dream is that it becomes a cornerstone on the way to a new and more global preventive medicine in the twenty-first century. Possible and obvious developments and by-products would be: thorough and modular checklists of risk factors as well as complete health promotion action plans for each disease/medical condition mentioned in this book and beyond.

Reference

Information included in this book was gathered from literally hundreds of Internet websites and articles, which were carefully selected following internationally recognized and renowned health institution guidelines or emanated from healthcare professionals with impeccable reputation and credentials. No single source was more prominent. Specific references are mentioned below tables

Chapter 2
Pointer Documents

2.1 Exercise

- Exercise increases HDL and decreases LDL and triglyceride levels. It also lowers blood pressure, reduces excess weight, improves heart and lung fitness, and diminishes stress.
- Engage in aerobic exercise (jogging, swimming, brisk walking, bicycling).
- As a rule, to be in aerobic conditions, one should be able to hold a conversation while exercising without being too winded.
- Recommended intensity: moderate. Moderate intensity is 5 or 6 on a 10-point scale of effort (from the Centers for Disease Control and Prevention).
- People are encouraged to wear pedometers to count the number of steps they take. Moderate intensity approximates 100 steps a minute.
- Adults are advised to accumulate 150 min of moderate-intensity aerobic activity every week in addition to strength training.
- Add strength training and flexibility to cardiovascular exercise.
- Lose weight before you exercise on a regular basis to avoid overload and resulting injuries on joints (particularly tendons).
- Start progressively.
- Be fit. How fit are you?

	Age	Unfit	Fit	Very fit
Men	20s	86 or more	60–85	59 or less
	30s	86 or more	64–85	63 or less
	40s	90 or more	66–89	65 or less
	50s and older	90 or more	68–89	67 or less
Women	20s	96 or more	72–95	71 or less
	30s	98 or more	72–97	71 or less
	40s	99 or more	74–98	73 or less
	50s and older	103 or more	76–102	75 or less

Y. Meunier, *Medicine of the Future: Risk Assessment, Elimination or Mitigation, and Action Plans for 28 Diseases and Medical Conditions*,
DOI 10.1007/978-3-319-07299-9_2, © Springer International Publishing Switzerland 2014

2.2   Stress Reduction

- Engage in generic stress reduction activities such as:

  - Meditation
  - Prayer
  - Laughter
  - Music
  - Reading
  - Massages
  - Sport (particularly martial arts)
  - Yoga
  - Tai chi
  - Shiatsu
  - Acupuncture
  - Acupressure

- Engage in specific stress reduction programs such as:

  - Reiki healing
  - Mindfulness-based stress management
  - HeartMath
  - Feldenkrais method
  - Biofeedback for stress management
  - Breathing to relax
  - Time management
  - Compassion, Awareness and Relationship Skills to Ease Stress (CARES)
  - Revitalize You! Online program to make your work-life work
  - From inside out. Effective ways to manage stress
  - Mind–body relaxation skills

Stress reduction includes *sleep improvement*. Various techniques are available to improve sleep quantity and quality, such as:

- Power Sleep®
- Sounder Sleep System®
- Calibrated exercise
- Hypnosis
- Acupuncture
- Yoga
- Reiki
- Shiatsu
- Massages

Sleep also affects body weight. People who sleep less often weigh more. Contact the Stanford Health Improvement Program for more information (http://hip.stanford.edu/).

2.3 Smoking Cessation

- The three-pronged approach is the most efficient one:
    1. Nicotine (to address physiological dependence)
    2. Bupropion (Zyban) (to address aggressiveness, bulimia)
    3. Psychological advice (for support and for determining the need behind the smoking habit)
- Ask your doctor to help you following the four A's rule (for him/her): Ask, Advise, Assist, and Arrange.
- Nicotine is not needed for less than ten cigarettes per day and contraindicated in case of drug interaction, in pregnant or breastfeeding women, and in teenagers.
- Nicotine inhaler or nasal spray is superior to patch.
- Ask your doctor about Chantix.
- Consider coaching programs.
- Consider Web-based programs.

2.4 Drink Standards and Recommendations (From the CDC)

A standard drink is equal to 14.0 g (0.6 oz) of pure alcohol. Generally, this amount of pure alcohol is found in:

- 12 oz of beer
- 8 oz of malt liquor
- 5 oz of wine
- 1.5 oz or a "shot" of 80-proof distilled spirits or liquor (e.g., gin, rum, vodka, or whiskey)

According to the *Dietary Guidelines for Americans*, moderate alcohol consumption is defined as having up to one drink per day for women and up to two drinks per day for men. This definition is referring to the amount consumed on any single day and is not intended as an average over several days.

The *Dietary Guidelines* also state that it is not recommended that anyone begin drinking or drink more frequently on the basis of potential health benefits because moderate alcohol intake also is associated with increased risk of breast cancer, violence, drowning, and injuries from falls and motor vehicle crashes.

2.5 Recommended Daily Amount of Fruits and Vegetables (From the CDC)

Please check the following website:
http://www.cdc.gov/nutrition/everyone/fruitsvegetables/howmany.html

2.6   Behavior Change

Behavior change is indispensable to get rid of deleterious lifestyles. Psychologists have studied human behavior for decades and proposed different models that would be efficient and sustainable.

The Stanford Health Improvement Program has created a science-based process that has proven to be manageable. It produces remarkable results and it is replicable and scalable.

2.6.1   3 Keys

- Self-management of lifestyle choices
- Selecting behaviors you are ready to change
- Setting realistic goals

2.6.2   15 Steps

1. Know your current behavior.
2. Assess readiness for change.
3. Gather knowledge.
4. Build a support network.
5. Make a commitment.
6. Set an appropriate long-term goal.
7. Set appropriate short-term goals.
8. Anticipate/deal with obstacles.
9. Manage stress.
10. Self-monitor.
11. Keep motivated.
12. Deal with ambivalence.
13. Cultivate a positive inner voice.
14. Be a mentor/opinion leader.
15. Reevaluate plan and adjust, if necessary.

2.6.3   Coaching

Behavior change is best achieved with a coach. He/she has a variety of tools to carry out his/her programs, such as face-to-face sessions, the Internet, telephone meetings, and social media (Twitter, Facebook, etc.), and make them as efficient as possible.

2.6.4   More Information

Please contact Dr. Deborah Balfanz:

- http://hip.stanford.edu/about/belfanz.html
- dbalfanz@stanford.edu
- 650-725-3185

2.7   Cholesterol Control Without Drugs

Please check the following webinar slides:
http://hip.stanford.edu/online-resources/Documents/Cholesterol%20
Presentation%20(2010).pdf

2.8   Preventing Diabetes

Please check the following webinar slides:
http://hip.stanford.edu/online-resources/Documents/Preventing_Diabetes_11-9-11.
pdf

2.9   Colorectal Cancer Prevention and Early Detection

Please check:

1. The following webinar slides:
   http://hip.stanford.edu/documents/Ladabaum%20CRC%20Webinar%20
   CCFZ%202010%20FINAL.pdf
2. The following video:
   http://www.youtube.com/watch?v=7dEKL3_0bYY

2.10   Breast Cancer

Please check the following slides:
http://www.cancer.org/acs/groups/content/@editorial/documents/document/
breast_cancer_powerpoint_packa.pdf

2.11   Prostate Cancer

Please check the following slides:
http://www.cancer.org/acs/groups/content/@editorial/documents/document/prostatecancerpowerpoint20pack.pdf

2.12   Lung Cancer

Please check the following slides:
http://www.cancer.org/acs/groups/content/@editorial/documents/document/prostatecancerpowerpoint20pack.pdf

2.13   Stomach Cancer

Please check the following website:
http://www.cancer.org/cancer/stomachcancer/detailedguide/index

Appendices

Other Books with the Same Author

Tropical Diseases: A Practical Guide for Medical Practitioners and Students

New York, Oxford University Press, 2013
http://global.oup.com/academic/product/tropical-diseases-9780199997909;jsessio
nid=68E89B0C7980B4040A54563708E8F419?cc=us&lang=en&

Tropical Diseases: 20 Case Studies

Los Gatos, Robertson Publishing, 2012
http://rp-author.com/meunier/

Global Health: Welcome to the Unexpected

Los Gatos, Robertson Publishing, 2011
http://rp-author.com/meunier/

Main Common and Tropical Diseases

Co-author, Paris, "Encyclopedie Jeune Afrique", fourth volume, 1980
http://www.worldcat.org/title/encyclopedie-ja-de-la-famille/oclc/84616164&referer=
brief_results

Y. Meunier, *Medicine of the Future: Risk Assessment, Elimination or Mitigation,* 139
and Action Plans for 28 Diseases and Medical Conditions,
DOI 10.1007/978-3-319-07299-9, © Springer International Publishing Switzerland 2014

Chagas Disease

In "Medecine Tropicale" by Marc Gentilini and Bernard Duflo. Contributing author,
Paris, Flammarion, fourth edition, 1986
    http://www.worldcat.org/title/medecine-tropicale/oclc/799266239/
editions?start_edition=11&sd=asc&referer=di&se=yr&editionsView=true&fq=

Health Assessments for Reduced Risk and Real ROI:
Innovations, Interventions and Incentives

Co-author with Gary Smithson, and Wes Alles. Sea Girt, Healthcare Intelligence
Network publishers, 2008
http://www.amazon.com/Health-Assessments-Reduced-Risk-Real/dp/193464756X

A Crucial Role for Health Promotion in the 21st Century

Foreword. Boca Raton, Annals of Medicine and Healthcare Research, Universal
Publishers, BrownWalker Press, 2009
 http://www.bookpump.com/bwp/pdf-b/942908Xb.pdf

Two Articles by the Same Author

Healthcare: The Case for the Urgent Need and Widespread Use of Preventive Medicine in the U.S.

Keywords

Cost-effectiveness, intervention, medicine, preventive, U.S.

Citation

Y Meunier. *Healthcare: The Case for the Urgent Need and Widespread Use of
Preventive Medicine in the U.S.* The Internet Journal of Healthcare Administration.
2008 Volume 6 Number 2.

Abstract

The cost of healthcare is ballooning in the U.S. with no end in sight to the trend despite the fact that we know how to limit and decrease it through preventive medicine. To reverse this non-sensible and soon-to-be unsustainable situation, this paper reiterates why preventive medicine is the best solution to control expenditure and improve mortality and morbidity across the board. It analyses different medical conditions and corporate interventions to make the case de novo at a crucial time and outlines some major obstacles to change. The author calls for prompt and drastic action in the form of a prevention Marshall-like national plan with information mass campaigns.

Background

The cost of curative medicine is constantly increasing in the United States with no foreseeable improvement. It has already reached staggering levels. The main causes of mortality are attributable to diseases, which are in various proportions preventable by lifestyle modifications. In 2005, 58.4 % of the major killers were in this category as follows [1, 2]:

(1) heart diseases (26.6 %), (2) cancer (22.8 %), (3) stroke (5.9 %), and (6) diabetes (3.1 %). For type 2 diabetes alone [3], the 2002 costs were sizable:

- Direct medical expenditure: $91.9 billion, divided as follows:

  - $23.2 billion for diabetes care
  - $24.6 billion for related chronic conditions
  - $44.1 billion for excess prevalence of general medical conditions

- Indirect expenditures: $39.8 billion, including the following:

  - Lost workdays
  - Restricted activity days
  - Permanent disability
  - Mortality

According to economists, the trend is for a worsening of this picture. Healthcare spending was $2.1 trillion in 2006 or 16 % of the GDP [4], which is a 6.7 % increase over the 2004 spending. It is projected to reach 19.5 % of GDP by 2017 [5, 6].

Objective

The objective of this paper is to re-affirm with hard data that preventive medicine is the best way to avoid a health care crisis in the U.S. Not only preventive medicine makes sense to reduce mortality and morbidity, but also it provides a good return on investment for federal and state institutions as well as corporations and the individual [7, 8].

Methodology

The author made a review of the recent literature in order to determine the financial impact of preventive measures at the medical condition and corporate level.

Results

Savings per Medical Condition

Abdominal Aortic Aneurysm

Savings

- $14,000 to $20,000 per Quality Adjusted Life Year (QALY). QALY is a way of measuring disease burden, including both the quality and quantity of life lived, as means of quantifying the benefit of a medical intervention. The QALY model requires utility, independence, risk neutrality and behavior. It is based on the number of years of life that would be added by the intervention. Although sometimes debated, particularly versus HYE (Healthy-Years Equivalent) [9], it is one of the best tools available to measure the impact of an initiative [10–13].
- Average cost of the necessary preventive procedure: $45–60 per person.

Intervention

- One time screening by ultrasound for men 65–75 who have ever smoked

Alcohol Misuse

Savings

$4.30 for $1.00 invested, according to the trial for early alcohol treatment project [14, 15]

Intervention

Screening of all adults and providing counseling intervention in primary care settings

Aspirin Therapy

Savings

- $11,000 per QALY gained [16, 17]
- Cost for 81 mg/day (1 tab of baby aspirin): less than 50 cents per week

Intervention

- Discussing AAS prevention with adults at increased risk for coronary heart disease

Cervical Cancer

Savings

$11,830 per QALY saved (in year 2000 dollars) [18–20]

Intervention

Screening every woman sexually active with a cervix, as follows:

(a) PAP test (yearly), or
(b) Liquid based PAP test (every 2 years), or
(c) a or b + HPV DNA test (every 3 years)

　　After 70, if at least 3 tests were normal in the last 10 years or post hysterectomy: Stop screening (except if the latter was performed for cancer or pre-cancer).

　　If there was diethylstilbestrol (DES) exposure before birth or the patient is HIV + or immunodepressed: Continue screening.

Colorectal Cancer

Savings

Average cost-effectiveness ratios: $10,000 to $30,000 per life-year saved (in year 2000 dollars), compared to no screening [22, 23]

Intervention

Screening men and women over 50. One procedure can be chosen from the following recommended six options:

1. Fecal occult blood test or fecal immunochemical test (yearly)
2. Flexible sigmoidoscopy (every 5 years)
3. Fecal occult blood test or fecal immunochemical test (yearly) + sigmoidoscopy (every 5 years)
4. Double contrast barium enema (every 5 years)
5. Computed tomographic colonography (every 5 years)
6. Colonoscopy (every 10 years)

Diabetes (Type 2)

Savings

In year 1997, the cost per QALY for targeted screening at age 55 was $34,375 compared to no screening [24, 25].

Intervention

Screening adults with high blood pressure or hyperlipidemia

Healthy Diet

Savings

Benefit-to-cost ratios:

- $10.64/$1.00 for a food and nutrition education program in Virginia [26]
- $10.75/$1.00 in Iowa [27]

Intervention

Behavioral dietary counseling for adult patients with hyperlipidemia and other risk factors for cardiovascular disease and diet-related chronic disease

Hypertension

Savings

Reducing blood pressure from less than 140/90 mmHg to less than 130/85 mmHg in high-risk individuals would increase life expectancy by 16.5–17.4 years and decrease lifetime medical costs by $1,450 [28–30].

Intervention

Screening adults over 18 for high blood pressure

Immunization

Savings

Children/Adolescents

- The routine childhood vaccination program saves nearly $10 billion in direct medical costs and $43 billion in social costs for every birth cohort [31].
- For varicella, hospitalization costs declined from $85 to $22.1 million in 2002, which was the year of introduction of the vaccine [32].

    Adults
    Age 65 to 79: Medicare managed care plan for influenza immunization saves $80 per year, per vaccinated individual.

Intervention

Children/Adolescents
    See the CDC immunization tables [33].
    Adults
    One flu shot every year. For other vaccinations, see the CDC immunization tables [34].

Motor Vehicle Accidents

Savings

(a) Children

   From $24 to $69 per child. These costs are comparable with those of counseling for other prevention messages [35–37].
(b) Adults

   Nets cost savings: $330 per patient intervention [38].

Interventions

(a) Child safety seat counseling sessions (11 × 1.5 mn)
(b) Counseling trauma patients on the dangers of alcohol

Sexually Transmitted Diseases

Savings

$177 saved per patient (in year 2002 dollars) [39]

Intervention

Gonorrhea in urban emergency settings: Screening women over 15 and under 29 using urine-based NAAT (Nucleic Acid Amplification Tests).

Breast Feeding

Savings

1993–1994 data from the special supplementation nutrition program for women, infants, and children (WIC) in Colorado studying formula feeding vs. breast-feeding:

The latter saved $478 in WIC costs and Medicaid expenditures during the first 6 months of the infants' life [40].

Intervention

Prenatal and postpartum care

Folic Acid Supplementation

Savings

$5,000 per QALY [41]

Intervention

Prenatal and postpartum care

Tobacco Cessation in Pregnant Women

Savings

$6.00 are saved for each dollar spent on smoking cessation programs in pregnant women [42, 43].

Intervention

Smoking cessation program

Prenatal and Pregnancy Care

Savings

A universal screening would save $3.69 million and prevent 64.6 cases of pediatric HIV infection for every 100,000 pregnant women screened [44].

Intervention

HIV testing in pregnant women

Smoking Cessation

Savings

Smokers who stopped smoking reduce potential medical costs associated with cardiovascular disease by about $47 during the first year and $853 during the following 7 years [45, 46].

Intervention

Screening all adults for tobacco use and providing cessation intervention

Savings from Corporate Preventive Medicine Interventions

Review of 72 Articles

After reviewing 72 articles on the topic, Aldana found that for each dollar invested in 3–5 years, the return on investment (ROI) was about:

- $4.00 saved in health costs
- $5.00 saved by reducing absenteeism

10-Year Study of Employees in a Healthcare Setting [48]

- ROI (for each dollar invested)
  - $6.52 saved in health costs and sick leaves
- Intervention

Health risk assessment (HRA), newsletter, self-care book, self-directed change materials, workshops, financial incentives

1-Year Study of Employees and Retirees at Blue Shield of California [49]

- ROI (for each dollar invested)
  - $6.00 saved in health costs
- Intervention

HRA, newsletter, self-care book, self-directed change materials, nurse line, serial feedback

2-Year Study of Retirees and Spouses of Bank of America in California [50]

- ROI (for each dollar invested)
  - $5.96 saved in health costs
- Intervention

HRA, self-directed change materials, serial feedback

3-Year Study of Employees at Procter and Gamble in Cincinnati [51]

- ROI (for each dollar invested)
  - $6.75 saved in health costs
- Intervention

HRA, newsletter, self-care book, telephone coaching, workshops, nurse line

2.5-Year Study of Employees and Retirees of Chevron in San Francisco [52]

- ROI (for each dollar invested)
  - $6.42 saved in health costs
- Intervention

HRA, newsletter, telephone coaching, workshops

3-Year Study of Employees at Citibank [53]

- ROI (for each dollar invested)

  - $4.64 saved in health costs

- Intervention

  HRA, newsletter, self-care book, telephone coaching, workshops, nurse line, serial feedback

5-Year Study of Employees at Daimler Chrysler at 14 Sites in Michigan [54]

- ROI (for each dollar invested)

  - $212.00 saved annually in medical costs

- Intervention

  HRA, self-care book, self-directed change, workshops, financial incentive

Discussion

The first mention of preventive medicine goes back to the Greek civilization. Hippocrates the great physician of the 5th century B.C. classified causes of disease and identified behavior-related and therefore actionable factors such as irregular food intake, exercise and habits. Much more recently, in 1978 the Alma–Ata declaration [55] emphasized the importance of prevention to improve global health. Nevertheless, in 2008 the concept of prophylaxis has not penetrated the U.S. society in significant ways because of various obstacles. The data presented above clearly show that preventive medicine is the best way not only to improve mortality and morbidity in the U.S, but also to decrease healthcare costs. Hopefully, they will lay to rest the false debate about the cost-effectiveness of preventive medicine. Similarly to global warming this useless controversy is delaying the tough choices that must be made. Authors like David Brown spread counterproductive ideas in the mass media [56]. Unfortunately, he echoes a vast number of papers in the health economics literature based on macro-economic analyses contending that healthcare costs will continue to rise despite preventive medicine initiatives because they are driven by technology. Their arguments are flawed at least on two counts:

Morally, it is questionable to let people suffer when their ailments can be avoided.

Financially, most of the time they do not take into account the indirect costs of illness which far exceed direct cost [55].

Their economic argument is very damaging because business deciders read these papers much more than medical ones and it provides the core of the rationale that maintains the status quo in disease prevention, but inertia is quickly fading as an option. This literature addresses the following:

1. The supply side and affirms that technological progress is the main driver for the observed healthcare cost continuous upward trend. It is obvious that a MRI procedure is much more expensive than an X-ray but it provides more information.

Therefore, it becomes more and more requested and performed. However, the need for both can be nullified if the patient stays in good health. Moreover, a broad debate needs to take place on the quality of care desired in the US and ways of better reimbursing prevention and strengthening the preventive supply side with incentives, in a general context. One option could be to move preventive care out of the medical realm into other societal spheres, keeping some medical oversight and guidance to be determined.

2. The demand side and questions the ability of prevention to raise welfare and maximize health. While it may be true that economical mathematics may show that total eradication of a plague in a society may not be the best goal to maximize health investments, the history of pandemics has proven otherwise in terms of global benefits.

Other authors [57, 58] warn that not all preventive medicine interventions will save money and recommend that careful analysis of the costs and benefits of specific interventions, rather than broad generalizations should be the rule. This analysis could identify not only cost-saving preventive measures but also delivering substantial health benefits relative to their net costs. Additionally, they suggest that it will be necessary to identify the preventive measures that are not yet fully deployed and those that could serve a large population and bring about significant overall improvements in health at an acceptable cost. Conversely, other services might be proven overused. These are common sense and general recommendations and most of these studies have already been carried out as this paper suggests. They clearly show that most preventive health interventions are cost-effective. By and large the obstacles to preventive medicine do not reside in the scientific community but rather in the mostly self-serving and ideological economic and political arenas.

Currently, the investment in the area of preventive medicine is minimal compared to the enormous needs. This includes federal, state, university, corporate, physician, and individual levels. Major obstacles toward prevention stand strong such as: The insurance, pharmaceutical industry, medical groups, food, agricultural and tobacco lobbies, to name a few. Analyses of deleterious cost spending by these entities are much needed, although data are often not available to the public and/or researchers. Despite hurdles on information gathering we know that, for example, from January 2005 through June 2006 alone, the pharmaceutical industry spent approximately $182 million on federal lobbying. This industry has 1,274 registered lobbyists in Washington DC [59].

It will take strong political will from the executive and legislative branches to turn the situation around. Moreover, it is unlikely to happen in the short term as their decisions would likely antagonize traditional political bases on both sides of the aisle if only by demanding or advocating for change and moving away from long lasting comfort zones. Sacrifices would be required without any previous national wide-scale experiment to refer to or with unwelcome models of preventive medicine and the way it is organized and implemented in countries like France, Canada and Great Britain [60]. Valuable lessons could be learned from their healthcare systems, in particular regarding immunization coverage and peri and pre-natal care. With the progressive increase in health insurance premiums, Americans are becoming more and more dissatisfied with the cost-effectiveness of their healthcare system [61].

This shift is not occurring in most single payer countries [62]. It seems that the solution starts with the fast and furious education of the masses. A huge paradigm shift is necessary, for example:

• While it is generally accepted that a vehicle in perfect working condition should get regular servicing to stay in good shape the same notion does not apply to human beings. Even for immunization, the following is interesting:

How many parents would have their children immunized if it were not mandatory to attend school?

How many adults keep their tetanus vaccination up to date every 10 years?

The acceptance of immunization was largely enabled by lethal epidemics. In these large events, scores of people were dying simultaneously. In 2008, the vast majority of people have long forgotten the following facts:

Poliomyelitis epidemics occurred in the US in 1894 (Vermont), in 1916 (widely spread), and between 1945 and 1949 (widely spread). In 1952, there were 58,000 cases and 35,000 in 1953. The baby boomer generation is the last one that grew up with the disease in its human environment and faced the dire consequences it carries. The subsequent generations are progressively forgetting the impact of the disease on a national and frequently personal level.

Diphtheria epidemics happened between 1735 and 1740 in the New England colonies. The mortality rate in children under 10 was as high as 80 %. In the 1920s, there were 100,000–200,000 cases a year with 13,000–15,000 deaths.

A pandemic of German measles epidemics took place between 1962 and 1965. In 1964–1965 the US had 12.5 million cases, which led to 11,000 miscarriages or therapeutic abortions and 20,000 cases of congenital rubella. Of these, 2,100 died as neonates, 12,000 were deaf, 3,580 blind and 1,800 mentally retarded.

Nowadays, hypertension, obesity and myocardial infarction (MI), to cite a few national and critical public health issues, affect many more people and differ because:

Deaths trickle in and do not happen concomitantly in mass.

They are not communicable diseases. Therefore, their threat is less acute. It must be noted however that obesity, for example, may spread like an infectious disease, the agent being food and drinks and the vector the feeding culture transmitted from one individual to another by families, friends, the media and culture of the susceptible individual.

They evolve on a chronic mode and are endemic. Even if MI is an acute event, it results from the slow buildup of the plaque.

When someone dies from MI, it is perceived more as an individual and internal tragedy (heart problem). When someone dies from diphtheria, it is seen more as an external and collective scourge (the spreading of a deadly bacterium). Hence, it becomes easier for society to mobilize against this common enemy.

Now that the threat of a "classic" infectious disease has vanished, people focus on the side effects of vaccines. The mass media, mainly for economic purposes, sometimes foments a negative image of this preventive intervention, reporting, for example, that the measles shot induces autism or that the hepatitis B vaccine causes multiple sclerosis. Doctors know the impact of such best-selling stories with increasing numbers of patients refusing to be vaccinated or turning to alternative medicine, which is highly inefficient in this regard. These facts on immunization illustrate how a highly efficient preventive medicine measure can become taken for granted and undervalued by a population.

- While certain preventive measures like stem cell or gene therapy are welcome and anxiously awaited, behavioral modifications are not so popular to prevent or delay the onset of a disease. Multiple economic, psychological and societal factors can explain the difference: Stress, instant gratification, availability of unhealthy agents almost everywhere, aggressive marketing, wrong role models, majority as the norm, etc

One must be aware of three facts: (1) the free market is inefficient at the national preventive medicine level because firms in the related trade would be depending on too many parameters to emerge (social, psychological, medical, economical, financial, political, national, international) and require massive investment in a pioneer field. Some companies are successful but have very limited impact offering, for example, exercise centers and wellness programs. However, no multifaceted proactive health corporation is currently represented at NYSE Euronext, (2) the same free market may be dangerous as seen on the internet with deviant medical practices promoted in the name of well-being. As a result, the new preventive medicine educational movement should be kept under some supervision of medical authorities, and (3) in order to obtain wide-spread societal behavioral change there should be short term benefits if they are adopted and/or negative consequences if they are denied. These could be determined and created at all levels.

Ultimately, the question remains: How can this massive transition be accomplished?

A task force encompassing all the partners and representing a cross-section of the American society could be nominated at the federal level to indicate the best action plan and strategies to move forward with an aggressive and ambitious agenda. It could take the form of a domestic Marshall-like plan aimed at saving the U.S. health care services by adapting them better to the current and future needs and based on preventive medicine. This would also be the opportunity for the States to become a leader in a new form of healthcare and spearhead innovative and economical solutions for challenges ahead.

Additional answers to this question and action are required promptly as the current dynamics are leading us to an unsustainable picture in human and treasure cost in the near future.

Conclusion

Preventive Medicine is vastly underutilized in the U.S. at a time when health costs are getting exorbitant and seemingly uncontrollable. However, it represents a very powerful, cost-effective and morally correct tool that can be used to avoid the looming health care crisis and improve the longevity and quality of life. In order to succeed radical action is needed at many levels without any delay.

Correspondence To

Yann A. Meunier, MD Health Promotion Manager Stanford Health Improvement Program Stanford School of Medicine Hoover Pavilion, N151 211 Quarry Road Stanford, CA 94305–5705 or: ymeunier@stanford.edu

References

1. Hsiang-Ching Kung et al (2008) National vital statistics reports. CDC 56(10):3
2. Mokdad AH, Marks JS, Stroup DF, Gerberding JL (2004) Actual causes of death in the United States, 2000. JAMA 291:1238–1245
3. Economic costs of diabetes in the U.S. in 2002 (2003) Diabetes Care 26(3):917–932
4. National Health Expenditure Data. NHE fact sheet, 26 Feb 2008
5. Keehan S et al (2008) Health spending projections through the baby boom generation is coming to medicare health affairs, web exclusive, 26 Feb 2008
6. Maciosek MV, Coffield AB, Edwards NM, Flottemesch TJ, Goodman MJ, Solberg LI (2006) Priorities among effective clinical preventive services: results of a systematic review and analysis. Am J Prev Med 31:52–61
7. Russell LB (2007) Prevention's potential for slowing the growth of medical spending. National Coalition on Health Care, Washington, DC
8. Weinstein MC (1999) High-priced technology can be good value for money. Ann Intern Med 130:857–858
9. Ried W (1998) QALY vs HYEs. What's right and what's wrong: a review of the controversy. J Health Econ (17):607–625
10. Silverstein MD, Pitts SR, Chaiko EL, Ballard DJ (2005) Abdominal aortic aneurysm: cost-effectiveness of screening, surveillance of intermediate sized AAA, and management of symptomatic AAA. Proc (Barl Univ. Medical Center) 12(4):345–367
11. Meenan RT, Fleming C, Whitlock EP, Beil TL, Smith P (2005) Cost-effectiveness analyses of population-based screening for abdominal aortic aneurysm: evidence synthesis. AHRQ electronic newsletter, vol 159. Agency for Healthcare Research and Quarterly, Rockville
12. Multicentre Aneurysm Screening Study Group (2002) Multicentre aneurysm screening study (MASS): cost effectiveness analysis of screening for abdominal aortic aneurysm based on four years results from a randomized controlled trial. BMJ 325:1135–1138
13. Lee TY, Korn P, Heller JA et al (2002) The cost-effectiveness of a "quick-screen" program for abdominal aortic aneurysms. Surgery 132(2):399–407
14. Fleming MF, Mundt MP, French MT, Manwell LB, Stauffacher EA, Barry KL (2002) Brief physician advice for problem alcohol drinkers: long-term efficacy and benefit-cost analysis. A randomized controlled trial in community-based primary care settings. Alcohol Clin Exp Res 26:36–43
15. Bertholet N, Daeppen JB, Fleming M, Burnand B (2005) Reduction of alcohol consumption by brief alcohol intervention in primary care: systematic review and meta-analysis. Arch Intern Med 165:986–95
16. Pignone M, Earnshaw S, Tice JA, Pletcher MJ (2006) Aspirin, statins, or both drugs for the primary prevention of coronary heart disease events in men: a cost-utility analysis. Ann Intern Med 144(5):326–336

17. Gaspoz JM, Coxson PG, Goldman PA, Williams LW, Kuntz KM, Hunink MGM, Goldman L (2003) Cost effectiveness of aspirin, clopidogrel, or both for secondary prevention of coronary heart disease. N Engl J Med 348(6):560

18. Mandelblatt JS, Lawrence WF, Womack SM, Jacobson D, Bin YI, Yi-Ting H et al (2002) Benefits and costs of using HPV testing to screen for cervical cancer. JAMA 287(18): 2372–2381

19. Brown ML, Lipscomb J, Snyder C (2001) The burden of illness of cancer: economic cost and quality of life. Ann Rev Public Health. 22:91–113

20. Eichler H, Kong SX, Gerth WC, Mavros P, Jensson B (2004) Use of cost-effectiveness analysis in health-care resource allocation decision-making: how are cost-effectiveness thresholds expected to emerge? Value Health 7(5):518–528

21. Swensen AR, Birnbaum HG, Secnik K, Marynchenko M, Greenberg P, Claxtion A (2003) Attention-deficit/hyperactivity disorder: increased costs for patients and their families. J Am Acad Child Adolesc Psychiatry 42(12):1415–1423

22. Taplin SH, Barlow W, Urban N, Mandelson MT, Timlin DJ, Ichikawa L et al (1995) Stage, age, comorbidity, and direct costs of colon, prostate, and breast cancer care. J Natl Cancer Inst 87(6):417–426

23. Pignone M, Saha S, Heorgem T, Mandelblatt J (2002) Cost-effectiveness analyses of colorectal cancer screening: a systematic review. Ann Intern Med 137:96–104

24. Diabetes Prevention Research Group (2003) Costs associated with the primary prevention of type 2 diabetes mellitus in the Diabetes Prevention Program. Diab Care 26:36–37

25. Hoerger TJ, Harris R, Hicks KA, Donahue K, Sorenson S (2004) Screening for type 2 diabetes mellitus: a cost-effective analysis. Ann Intern Med 140:689–710

26. Lambur M, Rajgopal R, Lewis Cox RH, Ellerbrock M (1999) Applying cost benefit analysis to nutrition education programs: focus on the Virginia Expanded Food and Nutrition Education Program. U.S. Department of Agriculture, Washington, DC

27. Wessman C, Betterley C, Jensen H. Evaluation of the costs and benefits of Iowa's Expanded Food and Nutrition Education Program (EFNEP): final report. Available from http://ideas.repec.org/p/ias/cpaper/01-sr93.html

28. Franco OH, Peeters A, Bonneux L, de Laet C (2005) Blood pressure in adulthood and life expectancy with cardiovascular disease in men and women: life course analysis. Hypertension 46:280

29. Fischer MA, Avorn J (2004) Economic implications of evidence-based prescribing for hypertension: can better care cost less? JAMA 291:1850–1856

30. Johannesson M, Jonsson B (1992) A review of cost-effectiveness analyses of hypertension treatment. Pharmacoeconomics 1:250–264

31. Zhou F, Santoli J, Messonnier ML, Yusuf HR, Shefer A, Chu SY et al (2005) Economic evaluation of the 7-vaccine routine childhood immunization schedule in the United States, 2001. Arch Pediatr Adolesc Med 159:1136–1144

32. Zhou F, Harpaz R, Jumaan AO, Winston CA, Shefer A (2005) Impact of varicella vaccination on health care utilization. JAMA 294:797–802

33. Centers for disease control and prevention (2007) MMWR Weekly 56(41)

34. Centers for disease control and prevention (2008) MMWR Weekly 57(01)

35. Walensky RP, Weinstein MC, Kimmel AP, Seage III GR, Losina SD, Zhang PE, Smith HE, Freedberg KA, Paltiel AD (2005) Routine human immunodeficiency virus testing: an economic evaluation of current guidelines. Am J Med 118:292–300

36. Ekwueme DU, Pinkerton SD, Holtgrave DR, Branson BM (2003) Cost comparison of three HIV Counseling and testing technologies. Am J Prev Med 25(2):112–121

37. Varghese B, Peterman TA (2001) Cost-effectiveness of HIV counseling and testing in U.S. prisons. J Urban Health 78(2):304–312

38. Gentilello L, Ebel B, Wickizer T, Salkever D, Rivara F (2005) Alcohol interventions for trauma patients treated in emergency departments and hospitals: a cost-benefit analysis. Ann Surg 241(4):541–550

39. Aledort JE, Hook III EW, Weinstein MC, Goldie SJ (2005) The cost-effectiveness of gonorrhea screening in urban emergency departments. Sex Transm Dis 327(7):425–436

40. Montgomery DL, Splett PL (1997) Economic benefit of breast-feeding infants enrolled in WIC. J Am Diet Assoc 97:379–385

41. Kelly AE, Haddix AC, Scanlon KS, Helmick CG, Mulinare J (1996) Cost-effectiveness of strategies to prevent neural tube defects. In: Gold MR, Siegel JE, Russell LB, Weinstein MC (eds) Cost-effectiveness in health and medicine. Oxford University Press, New York/Oxford, p 312–349

42. U.S. Public Health Service (2000) Treating tobacco use and dependence: a systems approach. Office of the U.S. Surgeon General/U.S. Public Health Service/U.S. Department of Health and Human Services, Rockville

43. Marks JS, Koplan JP, Hogue CJR et al (1990) A cost-benefit/cost-effectiveness analysis of smoking cessation for pregnant women. Am J Pre Med 6:282–291

44. Immergluck LC, Cull WL, Schwatrz A, Elstein AS (2000) Cost-effectiveness of universal compared with voluntary screening for human immunodeficiency virus among pregnant women in Chicago. Pediatrics 105(4):E54

45. Lightwood JM, Glantz S (1997) Short-term economic and health benefits of smoking cessation. Circulation 96(4):1089–1096

46. Warner KE, Smith RJ, Smith DG, Fries BE (1996) Health and economic implications of a work-site smoking-cessation program: a simulation analysis. J Occup Environ Med 38(10): 981–992

47. Aldana SG (2001) Financial impact of health promotion programs: a comprehensive review of the literature. Am J Health Promotion 15(5):296–320

48. Chapman L, Burt R, Fry J, Washburn J, Haack T, Rand J, Plankenhorn R, Brachet S Ten-year economic evaluation of an incentive-based worksite health promotion program. Am J Health Promotion, in publication

49. Fries JF, McShane D (1998) Reducing need and demand for medical services in high-risk persons. West J Med 169(4):201–207

50. Fries JF, Bloch D, Harrington H, Richardson N, Beck R (1993) Two-year results of a randomized controlled trial of a health promotion program in a retiree population. Am J Med 94:455–462

51. Goetzel RZ, Jacobson BH, Aldana SG, Vardell K, Yee L (1998) Health care costs of worksite health promotion participants and non-participants. J Occup Environ Med 40(4):341–346

52. Goetzel RZ, Dunn RL, Ozminkowski RJ, Satin K, Whitehead D, Cahill K (1998) Differences between descriptive and multivariate estimates of the impact of Chevron corporation's health quest program on medical expenditures. J Occup Environ Med 40(6):538–545

53. Ozminkowski RJ, Dunn R, Goetzel R, Cantor R, Murnane J, Harrison M (1999) A return on investment evaluation of the Citibank N.A. health management program. Am J Health Promot 14(1):32–43

54. Serxner SA, Gold DB, Grossmeir JJ, Anderson DR (2003) The relationship between health promotion program participation and medical costs: a dose response. J Occup Environ Med 54(11):1196–1200

55. "Les soins de sante primaires". Declaration d'Alma-Ata (1978) OMS-FISE, Geneve, (available in English)

56. Brown D (2008) In the balance, The Washington Post, 8 Apr 2008

57. Sullivan S (2008) Is treating disease cheaper than preventing it? An ounce of prevention is still worth a pound of cure. Inst Health Prod Manag. 2(1), editorial

58. Cohen JT, Neumann PJ, Weinstein MC (2008) Does preventive care save money? Health economics and the presidential race. N Engl J Med 358(7):661–663

59. Asif Ismail M (2007) Spending on lobbying thrives. Drug and health products industries invest $182 million to influence legislation. Report from the Center for Public Integrity, funded by the Nathan Cummings Foundation

60. Nathanson CA (2007) Disease prevention as social change: the state, society and public health in the Unites States, France, Canada and Great Britain. Russell Sage Foundation Publications

61. "Les services publics vus par les usagers", BVA actualite (2004) Le Point, 16 Sept 2004

62. ABCNews/Washington Post poll, 9–13 Oct 2003. http://abcnews.go.com/sections/living/us/healthcare031020_poll.html

What's New with Health Risk Assessments?

Keywords

Assessment, health, perspectives, risk, update

Citation

Y Meunier. *What's new with health risk assessments?* The Internet Journal of Health. 2007 Volume 8 Number 1.

Abstract

After briefly reviewing the historical background of health risk assessments (HRAs) and showing their recent renewed interest, the article discusses conditions for their effectiveness and exemplifies the return on investment they can yield. Finally, it outlines some future trends in the possible place of HRAs in preventive medicine at the individual and collective levels.

Introduction

Health risk assessments (HRAs) have been used for many years as a means to evaluate disease risks linked to lifestyle. With the de novo interest in preventive medicine in the U.S. an update on their use, value and perspectives seems timely.

Background

The first mention of the interaction between lifestyle and disease prevention goes back to the Greek civilization. Hippocrates, the great physician of the 5th century B.C., classified causes of disease and identified behavior-related and therefore actionable factors such as irregular food intake, exercise and habits.

Much more recently, in 1978 the Alma–Ata declaration [1] emphasized the importance of prevention to improve global health. Over the past forty years, there has been a growing awareness of the link between lifestyle and many major diseases, particularly in developed countries. Concomitantly, the exponential growth in costs associated with medical care has revived the interest in health risk appraisals in the United States.

HRAs were developed by Dr. Lewis Robbins [2] and first used in conjunction with the Framingham study. Their original purpose was to assess mortality risk. Then, this instrument evolved and led to the Geller tables [3] which were designed for primary care physicians with the same intent. The LaLonde Report [4] issued by the Canadian government in 1974 gave impetus to the perceived value of prospective medicine and stimulated interest by the Centers for Diseases Control, which developed its own HRA [5]. It included information on demographics, medical history and lifestyle behavior. Some other HRAs also incorporated clinical and biological data such as BMI, cholesterol and blood pressure to compute a health score. In the past thirty years HRSs had been in limbo. However, in the past three years approximately, a new focus has been found in HRAs' potential as a tool for education and behavior change.

In 2006, 19 % of employers with 500 or more employees offered incentives for HRAs compared to 7 % in 2004 [6]. In 2007, 91 % of employers believed they could reduce health costs by influencing healthier lifestyles [7]. In the same year, 66 % of insurers said they were somewhat or very likely to provide incentives for health-enhancing behaviors. Nevertheless, the vast majority of the economic literature concludes that preventive medicine is not cost-effective [8]. This evidence was drawn from macroeconomic analyses showing that the cost of healthcare is driven essentially by technology. As a matter of fact, many employers still consider wellness programs as benefits. Hence the value of preventive medicine which directly results in the reduction of use of all diagnostic devices.

This rekindled interest in HRAs and wellness programs is understandable since lifestyle accounts for about 50 % of mortality overall in the U.S. Furthermore, according to the MacArthur Foundation Select Panel on Healthy Aging, 80 % of health is determined by lifestyle in adults.

Discussion

In 2008, HRAs are used in isolation or followed up with different interventions: Health risk and reduction sessions, group coaching, one-on-one coaching, wellness programs, health education plans, and preventive medicine actions (e.g., immunization, screening, etc). These take place in a worksite, through a health plan, in a community clinic or in a general community-based program. HRAs are given with or without incentives. It is important to note that the failure of many wellness programs is due to the lack of a crucial step, which is the participant's motivation assessment. As an example, the Stanford science-based six-step method for behavior change [9] has been proven effective. It includes the following, with a variety of assessments and steps:

- Identifying the problem and assessing your current behaviors (healthy lifestyle behaviors vs. risks)
- Building confidence and commitment, assessing readiness for change and motivational assets (motivational assets available vs. those which need to be strengthened) and building a support network (who can help/what type of support they can provide/what is not needed from them)
- Increasing awareness of the behavior and keeping track of the behavior change progress
- Developing and implementing an action plan, setting a long-term goal (which must be sustainable and realistic), anticipating barriers and designing strategies

to overcome them, maintaining motivation (through benefits from the wellness plan and extrinsic rewards) and setting the first short-term goal (it has to be specific in time and part of a gradual progress)

- Evaluating the action plan and assessing motivation on a scale from 1 to 5 (if the score is less than 4, the goal must be re-visited)
- Maintaining the behavior change and preventing relapse by becoming an opinion leader and/or mentor, for example:

High participation to HRAs and health promotion programs is essential to yield a good return on investment. The conditions for high participation include: Good program (capturing interests, educating, encouraging behavior change), good communication plan starting from the top (e.g., CEO blast e-mails), easy navigation and understandability, easy accessibility (intranet, website), easy and fast completion (less than 15 min), adequate financial incentives and prizes, privacy, quality of output (in particular, quality of the aggregate report), quality of customer service (reputable and trusted provider).

Participation has been proven much lower without financial incentives. On average, with a $100 incentive a 66 % participation can be achieved. Other material incentives include, for example: gift cards, merchandise, health club membership, health account contribution [10], sport items (bicycles, tennis rackets, running shoes), etc.

The main issues of concern to potential participants in HRAs encompass legal matters [11] (in particular, privacy and Health Insurance Portability and Accountability Act or HIPAA).

Summary

- HRAs are more commonly used than ever in 2008.
- Their quality varies greatly. Good ones are science-based.
- Participation is much higher with financial incentives [10].
- Best results are achieved when HRAs are followed by health promotion/wellness programs [7].
- Good return on investment is achieved with the right program design and implementation.
- There is (a) cumulative effect and (b) dose response [12–14].

The cumulative effect means that the result produced by two different health promotion interventions is greater than the sum of them considered separately. This is due in part to the fact that health awareness in these two domains reverberates onto other healthy behaviors by osmosis. The dose response implies that the higher the number of participants the better the results [15, 16]. Several studies have demonstrated significant return on investment (on average $5.75 for $1.00) after using HRAs as the basis for health promotion interventions. They are shown in the following synthesis made by the author:

Fig. 1 Return on investment from health promotion programs. From: "HRAs and ROI." http://www.powershow.com/view/b0c1c-OTYxY/HRAs_and_ROI_powerpoint_ppt_presentation

Source	Health Costs ROI (for $1.00)
Review of 72 Articles	$4.00
Health Care Setting	$6.52
Blue Shield, CA	$6.00
Bank of America, CA	$5.96
Procter & Gamble, OH	$6.75
Chevron, CA	$6.42
Citibank	$4.64

Another 5-year study conducted among employees of Chrysler Daimler Benz in 14 sites in Michigan showed an average $212.00 annual return on each $1.00 invested [24]. In his review, Pelletier found that from 2000 to 2004, the vast majority of more than 122 research studies to date indicated positive clinical and cost outcomes [25]. Moreover, often this return on investment happens within the first year of intervention [26].

Future Trends of HRAs

In the near future, HRAs have a great potential in advancing the agenda of preventive medicine. For example:

(a) *Medical conditions*

Currently, health promotion interventions are focusing on lifestyle modification to stop smoking, decrease weight, exercise sufficiently, reduce stress, eat in a healthy way, screen for cancer, or update immunizations. However, going forward new fields may be included such as early detection of medical conditions and preventive therapy such as, for example:

• *Abdominal aortic aneurysm*

Savings

$14,000 to $20,000 per Quality Adjusted Life Year [27]. Quality-Adjusted Life Year (or QALY) is a way of measuring disease burden, including both the quality and the quantity of life lived, as a means of quantifying in benefit of a medical intervention. The QALY model requires utility, independence, risk neutrality and behavior. It is based on the number of years of life that would be added by the intervention.

Intervention

One time screening by abdominal ultrasound for men 65–75 who have ever smoked (average cost, $45–60 per person)

- *Aspirin therapy*

Savings

$11,000 per QALY gained

Intervention

Discussing aspirin prevention with adults at increased risk for coronary heart disease (cost, 81 mg/day, which amounts to less than 50 cents/week) [28]

(b) *Bridging the healthcare gaps*

Combining the HRA information with health data stemming from health plans, pharmacy drug use pattern, benefit/human resources department and medical parameters stored in electronic databases such as Microsoft Vault or Google Health, it will be possible to:

- Improve care management by creating real time care gap alerts.
- Determine a population health profile more accurately and comprehensively.
- Establish health priority needs and design tailored health promotion interventions.

(c) *Consultation tool*

- For physicians, the major obstacle to physician following up more actively on HRAs and health promotion programs is financial. Preventive medicine at the medical office level is not time-efficient, some may even say it is counterproductive. Another crucial issue is the assessment of a physician's preventive work. If a patient is given the knowledge and tools to adopt a healthy behavior, it is impossible to prove that, for example, a heart attack has been prevented. Therefore, how can physicians be remunerated fairly for their preventive medicine services? If medical practitioners are to play a more integrated and important role in the future in relation to HRAs, a compensation or incentive mechanism must be created in order to get their buy in. Increased use of HRAs would be an additional asset to them. For example, the summary report can serve as a data gathering tool by the physician.
- For patients, the HRA can serve as a communication tool as follows:

  - The introduction of a patient to a doctor
  - The basis of the doctor-patient relationship. For example, for requesting a wellness appointment
  - Being an instrument for teaching the patient how to become a better consumer

Conclusion

HRAs have been around for a long time and have evolved progressively. Recently, there has been a surge in their interest. This phenomenon is interesting for preventive medicine as a whole because when they are used adequately as the port of entry to health promotion programs they produce good return on investment and contribute significantly to health improvement. Furthermore, HRAs can be efficient tools for physicians and patients for improving the quality of medical services.

References

1. "Les soins de sante primaires". Declaration d'Alma-Ata (1978) OMS-FISE, Geneve, (available in English)
2. Robbins LC, Hall J (1970) How to practice prospective medicine. Methodist Hospital of Indiana, Indianapolis
3. Lang RS, Hensrud DD (2004) Clinical preventive medicine, American Medical Association, 2nd edn, chapter 42, p 477
4. http://www.hc-sc.gc.ca/hcs-sss/alt_formats/hpb-dgps/pdf/pubs/1974-lalonde/lalonde-eng-pdf
5. http://www.cdc.gov/NCCDPHP/dnpa/hwi/program_design/health_risk_appraisals.htm
6. National survey of employer-sponsored health plans: 2006 survey report (2007) Mercer Human Consulting, New York
7. Strategic health perspectives data sheet questionnaires 2007 (2007) Harris Interactive, New York
8. Brown D (2008) In the balance, The Washington Post, 8 Apr 2008
9. Farquhar J (1987) The American way of life need not to be hazardous to your health. Addison-Wesley publishing company
10. Heimes S (2008) Driving behavior change with interactive program. White paper. OptumHealth. OptumHealth.com
11. Michele M, Mello, Meredith B, Rosenthal (2008) Wellness programs and lifestyle discrimination- the legal limits. N Engl J Med 359:2
12. Sexner SA, Gold DB, Grossmeir JJ, Anderson DR (2003) The relationship between health promotion program participation and medical costs: a dose response. J Occup Environ Med 45(11):1196–2000
13. Scanes L, Coulson K (2002) A health promotion program for your workplace? Is it important and how will you know which one to choose? Queensland mining industry health & safety conference, 4–7 Aug 2002. Conference Proceedings, Townsville, p 61–68
14. Health risk appraisals address employees' individual problems: programs aim to instill healthy habits. Goliath Business Knowledge on Demand. Online, 2008
15. Vital studies in health promotion. Health enhancement systems. Online, 2008
16. Purdue health improvement initiative. Literature review. Online, 2008
17. Aldana SG (2001) Financial impact of health promotion programs: a comprehensive review of the literature. Am J Health Promot 15(5):296–320
18. Chapman L, Burt R, Fry J, Washburn J, Haack T, Rand J, Plankenhorn R, Brachet S. Ten-year economic evaluation of an incentive-based Worksite Health Promotion Program. Am J Health Promot, (in publication)
19. Fries JF, McShane D (1998) Reducing need and demand for medical services in high-risk persons. West J Med 169(4):201–207

20. Fries JF, Bloch D, Harrington H, Richardson N, Beck R (1993) Two-year results of a randomized controlled trial of a health promotion program in a retiree population: The Bank of America study. Am J Med 94:455–462

21. Goetzel RZ, Jacobson BH, Aldana SG, Vardell K, Yee L (1998) Health care costs of worksite health promotion participants and non-participants. J Occup Environ Med 40(4):341–346

22. Goetzel RZ, Dunn RL, Ozminkowski RJ, Satin K, Whitehead D, Cahill K (1998) Differences between descriptive and multivariate estimates of the impact of Chevron corporation's health quest program on medical expenditures. J Occup Environ Med 40(6):538–545

23. Ozminkowski RJ, Dunn R, Goetzel R, Cantor R, Murnane J, Harrison M (1999) A return on investment evaluation of the Citibank, N.A. health management program, Am J Health Promot 14(1):31–43

24. Serxner SA, Gold DB, Grossmeier JJ, Anderson DR (2003) The relationship between health promotion program participation and medical costs: a dose response. J Occup Environ Med 54(11):1196–1200

25. Pelletier KR (2005) A review and analysis of the clinical and cost-effectiveness studies of comprehensive health promotion and disease management at the worksite: update VI 2000–2004. J Occup Environ Med. 47:1051–1058

26. Bunn William B, Stave Gregg M et al (2006) Effect of smoking status on productivity loss. J Occup Environ Med. 48:1–10

27. Meenan RT, Fleming C, Whitloc EP, Beil TL, Smith P (2005) Cost-effectiveness analyses of population-based screening for abdominal aortic aneurysm: evidence synthesis. AHRQ electronic newsletter, vol 159. Agency for Healthcare Policy and Research, Rockville. Quarterly 4 Feb 2005

28. Pignone M, Earnshaw S, Tice JA, Pletcher MJ (2006) Aspirin, statins or both drugs for the primary prevention of coronary heart diseases in men: a cost-utility analysis. Ann Intern Med 144(5):326–336

Author's Information

Yann Meunier is a healthcare consultant based at Cochin Hospital in Paris, France.

He was the director of International Business Development and Public Affairs for Stanford Hospital and Clinics. At Stanford University, he was the director of the Stanford Health Promotion Network and a health promotion manager at the Stanford Prevention Research Center. He lectured at the University of California San Francisco. He was adjunct assistant professor of Medicine at George Washington University and assistant professor in public health at Paris VI University.

As the chief medical officer for a US corporation, he created and implemented a public health program for 10,000 villagers in the Kutubu area of Papua New Guinea. He led or participated in public health missions in Rio de Janeiro (Brazil), Montrouis (Haiti), Luanda (Angola), Casamance (Senegal), Ouesso (Republic of Congo), Port Harcourt (Nigeria), Lifou (New Caledonia), and the Yunnan Province of China.

LinkedIn Profile
http://www.linkedin.com/profile/view?id=3214361&trk=nav_responsive_tab_profile
Postal Address
8 Bd Jourdan
Paris 75014
France
E-mail Address
ymeuniermd@gmail.com

Printed in the United States
By Bookmasters